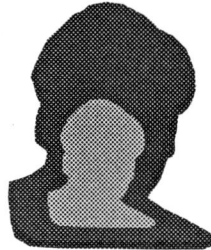

Person-Centred Care

Creative approaches to individualised care for people with dementia

Editor
Sue Benson

Foreword
Professor Bob Woods

Introduction and concept
Professor Tom Kitwood

THE JOURNAL OF DEMENTIA CARE
Person-Centred Care Series

PERSON-CENTRED CARE

Creative approaches to individualised care for people with dementia

This book draws together the Person-Centred Care series published
in the *Journal of Dementia Care*

First published in 2000 by
Hawker Publications Ltd
13 Park House
140 Battersea Park Road
London SW11 4NB
Tel 020 7720 2108, fax 020 7498 3023

British Library Cataloguing in Publication Data

A Catalogue in Publication Data

ISBN 1 874790 54 X

Designed by Andrew Chapman

Printed and bound by The Book Factory, London

Hawker Publications publishes *The Journal of Dementia Care*. For further information
please contact Hawker Publications at the address above or see our website: http://dementia.careinfo.org

Books published by Hawker Publications include:
Openings – Dementia Poems & Photographs. By John Killick and Carl Cordonnier. £9.99.
ISBN 1 874790 49 3. 2000.
Care to Communicate. By Jennie Powell. £16.95. ISBN 1 874790 48 5. 2000.
ASTRID – A guide to using technology within dementia care. Compiled and edited by Mary Marshall. £9.99.
ISBN 1 874790 52 3. 2000.
The Care Assistant's Guide to Working with People with Dementia.
Edited by Sue Benson. £13.50. ISBN 1 874790 37 X. 1998.
Improving Dementia Care: a resource for training and professional development.
By Buz Loveday, Tom Kitwood and Brenda Bowe. £59.99. ISBN 1 874790 38 8. 1998.
You Are Words – Dementia Poems. Edited by John Killick £6.50.
ISBN 1 874790 32 9. 1997, reprinted 2000.
Design for Dementia. Edited by Stephen Judd, Mary Marshall and Peter Phippen. £49.50.
ISBN 1 874790 35 3. 1997.
The New Culture of Dementia Care. Edited by Tom Kitwood and Sue Benson. £17.50.
ISBN 1 874790 17 5. 1995, reprinted 1997.

All books are available from Hawker Publications as above or
through reputable bookshops.

Contents

Contributors

CATHY CHATTEN wrote Chapter 11 while working as nurse researcher, Cardiff Community Healthcare. She is now a community nurse in north Yorkshire.

DEBBIE CHRISTIAN RMN is regional general manager for Care UK.

JOAN COSTELLO wrote Chapter 6 while working as head of home at Westbury, Methodist Homes for the Aged's specialist dementia care home.

FAITH GIBSON is emeritus professor in social work at the University of Ulster at Jordanstown, Belfast.

ANTHEA INNES worked as a part-time activities organiser in residential and nursing homes. She is now a researcher with Bradford Dementia Group.

MICHELLE JEFFERIES is a ward sister at Frenchay Hospital, North Bristol NHS Trust.

TOM KITWOOD was Alois Alzheimer Professor of Psychogerontology at the University of Bradford and leader of Bradford Dementia Group, until his death in 1998.

JO MARLEY co-wrote Chapter 1 while working as services director, Bryson House, Belfast.

HELEN MᶜVICKER co-wrote Chapter 1 while working as coordinator of the intensive domiciliary care team based in Shankill House, Belfast. She is now a lecturer in social work at the University of Ulster.

MARIE MILLS is a dementia care practitioner and researcher at the University of Southampton.

TRACY PACKER is consultant nurse in dementia care (acute services), North Bristol NHS Trust.

TRACY PETRE was a research psychologist with Bradford Dementia Group at the University of Bradford, until her death in 1996.

JACKIE POOL is a consultant occupational therapist in dementia care (Dementia Concern training and development practice).

GRAHAM STOKES is consultant clinical psychologist at Premier Health NHS Trust, Staffordshire, and consultant director of mental health, BUPA Care Homes.

MARGARET ANNE TIBBS is an independent consultant and trainer in dementia care, associated with Bradford Dementia Group and the Alzheimer's Society.

DR DAPHNE WALLACE wrote this chapter while working as consultant psychiatrist for the elderly, High Royds Hospital, West Yorkshire. Now retired, she works for the Alzheimer's Society as a volunteer.

BOB WOODS is professor of clinical psychology of the elderly, University of Wales, Bangor.

Foreword: Person-centred care – success stories?

BOB WOODS

What do we mean by success in caring for a person with dementia? It cannot mean reversing the irreversible – but, as Professor Bob Woods explores, it can be found in an individual, respectful and responsive approach.

The late Tom Kitwood wrote the introduction to this fascinating series of articles in the *Journal of Dementia Care* in 1995. The contributors were commissioned to produce 'success stories' – a detailed account of the story of one person with dementia with whom they had been involved – and these stories appeared in successive issues of JDC from Nov/Dec 1995 to the end of 1997. The aim was to challenge the notion that dementia must inevitably be characterised by decline, disintegration and despair. This would be achieved by highlighting the potential for improved well-being in situations where it proved possible to reverse the malignant social psychology; in effect, to rescue them from its crushing, devaluing, depersonalising power, about which Kitwood has written so eloquently (Kitwood 1997).

Reviewing the 13 case studies assembled here, it is impossible not to be struck by the limitations of our usual conceptions of 'success' in the context of dementia. There are certainly not many conventionally happy endings here to rejoice in. No one recovered from their dementia, or went back to their previous activities. The improvements documented are mainly concerned with reductions in disruptive behaviour, and it is of interest to note the prominence of such 'challenging' behaviour in these studies. Agitation, distress, withdrawal, hostility, aggression, violence, verbal abuse, punching, pinching, swearing, wandering, double incontinence, lack of compliance, screaming, kicking, scratching and biting all make an appearance at some point, and indeed represent a considerable challenge to the tolerance, resilience and coping ability of families and staff seeking to provide care.

In many of the case studies, such challenging behaviour did reduce, in at least one instance (3)* to a miraculous extent. It is important to be clear however that what is being described here is not simply a new approach to tackling aggression and the like in dementia, to render people with dementia more manageable, amenable and compliant, to reduce the strain and frustration borne by those stretched to the limit in an arduous care-giving task. Rather, the success recorded here in reducing challenging behaviour lies in the accompanying decrease in ill-being in the person with dementia, and the potential then apparent for an increase in the person's well-being and quality of life. Agitation and withdrawal both imply states of ill-being, with the person being overshadowed and obscured by their difficulties. In virtually every case, we see at some point the person becoming clearly present again, coming to the foreground, and some continuity with their 'old self' happily emerging.

In Chapter 4, Graham Stokes makes clear that it was not Mr D's behaviour which had changed, but rather other people's understanding of it. This served to contribute to a reduction in ill-being for Mr D to the extent that those around him were able to be less confrontational, and to prevent those aspects of his behaviour which created the most negative reactions in those with whom he came into contact. The limited nature of the success in this case is emphasised by the suggestion that it was the progression in Mr D's cognitive impairment which ultimately freed him from the powerful instinctual drive thought to underlie his behaviour, and which would not allow him peace of mind.

A reason for every behaviour?

The understanding of difficult and disruptive behaviour emerges as an important aspect in nearly every case. In the majority, this understanding comes from knowledge and awareness of the person's background and history, enabling a care plan to be established reflecting previous patterns of personal care and past preferences and interests. Listening to familiar music was important for Andy (1) and Elsie (10), but it is important to note that although Elsie had been a piano teacher, she would not now play a keyboard. Where a person feels their skills have declined, they may not wish to pursue a former interest at a lower level than previously enjoyed, and care needs to be taken to build on the person's interest in such a way so as not to expose them to failure. In some cases, recognition of aspects of the person's previous personality style was important: Ruby (11) enjoyed a good argument; George (5) was meticulous and precise; Mr D (4) was obsessional

Numbers in brackets refer to chapters in this book.

and a born worrier; Amos (3) was very religious; Elsie (10) was a solitary person; Mrs T (13) had a phobia regarding institutions (as well as toilet seats).

In a few cases, awareness of traumatic episodes in the person's past proved to be a key to understanding their current behaviour. Mrs O (8) had been sexually abused as a child, and now found personal care very distressing, unless carried out in a medical context. Being separated from her husband brought back painful memories of a previous wartime separation for Vera Browning (6). Mr D's behaviour (4) was seen as reflecting a traumatic incident he had experienced 15 years previously. The re-emergence of these traumatic memories, played out in behavioural disturbance, echoes Naomi Feil's conception of resolution of past memories, conflicts and 'unfinished business' in dementia (Feil 1993).

Current, unrecognised problems were also important in several instances. It is difficult for people with severe impairments to communicate the nature and extent of any pain experienced; in two cases (3 and 10), recognizing and treating the person's pain was an important aspect of the care plan. In chapter 13, recognition of the negative side effects of medication produced a rapid change in the person's ability when the medication was stopped. Attention to the person's physical health is an important component of person-centred care.

Attachment

Person-centred care is enriched when the person with dementia enjoys a close relationship with a significant person in their life. For Bessy (2), it was an attachment bond with the sheltered housing warden; for Amos (3), there were important relationships with his wife and with members of his community and church; for Vera Browning (6) and Andy (1), maintaining their relationship with their spouse was vital to their well-being; Fred's activity programme and its effects helped his son to see him as a person again (9). The relationship is not always with a person; it was only through Ruby's toy dog Toby that contact could be made (11); Mrs T (13) had a special teddy bear, and appeared to enjoy tactile contact; Elsie did not relate well to people, but spent hours stroking the ward cat, which sat contentedly on her lap. Perhaps these relationships offer the person with dementia more of an opportunity to contribute to the relationship, to offer affection without fear of rejection, especially where the person is generally not comfortable with intimacy. The relationship of Marie Mills and Amy (12) is described very much as a two-way exchange, with Marie reporting that she benefited greatly from their contacts, leaving her with a 'gift' of the memories of their shared experiences.

Similarly, Anthea Innes describes a special relationship with Mrs G (7), where Mrs G became her ally in setting up activities, and would rush to greet her when she arrived at the home. To allow a two-way relationship, for the person to be able to reciprocate, requires the caregiver to be open to receiving what the person with dementia is able to offer; many of us are so busy giving care that we do not recognise the opportunities for the person with dementia to fulfil their need to give care and affection.

An inadequate system?

Most of the cases were, at some stage of the story, in hospital or a residential/nursing home. For some, it seemed that they were caught within a system that was letting them down. Amos (3) was being looked after in what must have seemed to him to be an alien environment, having little to connect with his own culture and previous life. Ruby (11) and Mrs T (13) had both been the victim of multiple moves, triggering a spiral of disturbance and difficulty. Mrs T was restrained chemically and, with cot-sides at night, physically – only exacerbating her difficulties.

Anthea Innes considers that for Mrs G (7), a person-centred approach came too late, and that a different programme of care could have evolved if staff had appreciated how she had been before she came into the home. It was known that she would prefer a single room, but had to share, because a single room was not available. This added to her anguish at being in the home. It is difficult to follow a person's preferences and choices when they seem to place the person at risk, but as is clear with Ruby and with Amos, at times it is important to allow the person to follow their choice, while doing everything possible to reduce the danger of a negative consequence to a minimum.

It may be, of course, that the cases reported here are biased towards those where a person has been indeed 'rescued' from a malignant system, and there may be many more positive, responsive, flexible systems of care provision, such as that evident in chapter 12. However, many of us will recognise only too well how our well-meaning, well-intentioned systems so often let down the people they have been set up to serve.

A good death?

Several of the case studies end with the death of the person with dementia. Most occur in hospital, after the person has been admitted following a fall, or a chest infection. In most cases, there is a feeling that something positive and worthwhile had been achieved before the person died.

There is greater ambivalence in Anthea Innes'

description of Mrs G (7). While there had been indications of Mrs G's personhood breaking through in activity sessions, generally there was a sense that an understanding of her as a person came too late in her career as a person with dementia. Her prophetic words, that she could only leave the residential home in a coffin, proved ultimately to be essentially correct.

There is increasing realisation that the quality of a person's death is a vital component of their quality of life, but in most of these specific cases we cannot know how the final period of hospitalisation, be it days or weeks, was experienced by the person with dementia. We know that they were exposed to an unfamiliar environment, which most of us would find bewildering, and that they were struggling with the discomfort and probable pain of physical illness, which may well have added further to their confusion.

We can only hope that they were able to recognise the security and safety represented by the nurses in uniform, reassuring and confident in their nursing tasks, and that their pain and discomfort were recognised and alleviated. There is little doubt, however, regarding the quality of Ruby's death, as reported by Debbie Christian (11). She held tightly onto Debbie, reflecting the strength of their relationship which had been mediated initially through her beloved soft toy Toby, and died in her arms. Ruby had delighted in arguments with Debbie, as long as she emerged victorious, and found comfort with someone who had helped provide a sense of 'home' for a person who had been shunted between hospitals and homes previously. This really did seem to be a success.

Conclusion

It will be evident from these case studies that there is no one formula for 'success'. These cases are characterised by a highly individualized, respectful, flexible, responsive approach. Wherever possible, there has been a concern to maintain continuity with the person's past, to have an awareness and understanding of the person's life story and a sense of their identity. The person's other psychological needs (Kitwood 1997) – for comfort, attachment, social relations and occupation – have been evident, but above all these stories have been about the person with dementia having been accepted as a person, with the disturbed behaviour being seen as potentially understandable, as we discover more about the person and his/her circumstances.

In his introduction, Kitwood proposed that there could be three main explanations for success in these case studies:
• Individual differences in type and severity of neuropathology, so that success would occur with those with less neurological impairment.

• Variations in previous personality and life history, and thus resilience as persons in the face of neuropathological change.
• Positive outcomes are a direct consequence of the quality of care provided.

In reading these accounts, the impression emerges that it is the third of these possibilities which predominates. This is not altogether surprising, as most of the stories concern a turnaround in the person's well-being and/or function. These are not stories about people who are diagnosed as having dementia but whose cognitive impairment progresses slowly, if at all, or about those who maintain cheerful, positive roles and relationships in the face of their impairment.

Amy (12) might perhaps be an example of someone with a resilient personality, but even here the interaction of her coping and the person-centred care being offered is impressive. Certainly, there can be no suggestion that these people with dementia are less severely impaired than others, and the longitudinal aspect of most stories confirms the history of continuing impairment.

Can these stories be seen as examples of 'rementia'? They certainly support the notion that the person's presentation is not simply a function of the degree of neuropathological impairment. In a number of cases, people appeared more impaired because of the extent of distress, agitation, withdrawal or behavioural disturbance; when this was tackled, some of the excess disability was removed, and the person's presentation became a closer approximation to that consistent with the level of neuropathology. Other sources of excess disability, such as pain and medication were also evident. It would be difficult to conclude from the evidence here that the neuro-pathological impairments were reversed in any case, and the term 'rementia' might give a misleading impression of the process of change. Certainly, there is here further support for Kitwood's assertion that 'if the quality of care is good... there are beneficial effects for some'. These beneficial effects make more pressing and urgent the need to continually improve the quality of dementia care.

The longitudinal descriptions here remind us also that many of the transitions that occur in dementia care are not related to the person making some inevitable journey through the 'stages' of dementia. Many relate to changes in the care system; a family member becomes ill or has an accident, for example. Others are driven by the person's physical health: the person has a chest infection or a stroke. Behavioural disturbance does not automatically increase as dementia progresses, and as we have seen here, such disturbances may resolve. When they do occur they may in part be maintained by the care environment and the person's reaction to it.

Kitwood comments in his introduction: 'There is so much about personhood that we haven't grasped.' The case studies here add greatly to our practical understanding of the construct. There is the ethic of respect, that people with dementia are people of full human worth and value, despite their disability; but there is also here the indication that personhood finds its expression in relationship to another human being. It is not enough that we who are strong and intact provide care for the weak, frail and vulnerable; rather, we who have difficulty communicating with and understanding people with dementia, must seek to learn from them how to be fully human ourselves in listening and relating to them (Woods, 1999).

In these case studies, there are many glimpses of creative care workers placing themselves in this position, and at times succeeding in allowing the personhood of the person with dementia to emerge and even flourish. We owe them gratitude for pointing the way forward for us all. Clearly, as Kitwood predicted, 'some of the anguish and sorrow that surrounds dementia is beyond our power to take away'. But here there are insights that 'shine like a jewel in the light'. I hope they will inspire many more to discover person-centred care and to record and share their experiences.

References

Feil N (1993) *The Validation breakthrough: simple techniques for communicating with people with "Alzheimer's type dementia"*. Health Professions Press, Baltimore.

Kitwood T (1997) *Dementia reconsidered: the person comes first*. Open University Press, Buckingham.

Woods B (1999) The person in dementia care. *Generations* 23(3) 35-39.

Introduction: Building up the mosaic of good practice

TOM KITWOOD

The stories now collected in this book, which were originally published in the *Journal of Dementia Care*, are an important preliminary to the formal research on care practice which is vitally needed if our knowledge of dementia care is to advance, Tom Kitwood argues.

Slowly and steadily, year by year, our knowledge about how to care well for people with dementia is growing. As each new discovery is made, it is as if we are finding the different pieces that make up a vast mosaic; and as we begin to fit them together, a beautiful, elaborate and mysterious pattern is taking shape.

Some of the individual pieces of this mosaic are now fairly well known: for example, the use of validation and reminiscence, or the requirements for making a place feel homely, comfortable and reassuring. Other pieces are less familiar, and we are still exploring their shape and colour: for example, how to provide good stimulation for the senses, or how to enable each individual to find his or her own expressive language even when the powers of speech have failed. I am sure that many pieces of the full mosaic are yet to be discovered. After all, there is so much about personhood that we haven't grasped, as well as all that we don't know about dementia.

The heart of person-centred care

What lies at the heart of the approach that is coming to be called person-centred care? As I understand it, there are two main ingredients, intimately mixed together: an ethic and a social psychology.

The ethic asserts, as a statement that is beyond challenge, that all human beings have absolute value, regardless of how "good" or "bad", how able or disabled, they may be. We thus have an obligation to treat each other with deep respect: as ends, and never as means to some other end. The ethic can be accepted simply as the only assumption on which our existence as social beings, endowed with the capacity both to love and to suffer, makes sense; it also harmonises with the highest moral codes found in each of the main religions and spiritual paths (see, for example, Mackie (1983) and Post (1996).

The second ingredient – the social psychology – is a body of knowledge which shows in detail how people with dementia can live out their lives in the most fulfilling way (maintaining relationships, exercising choice, experiencing satisfaction, and so on). For that knowledge to be sound, it must be well tested. It will also be compatible with the genuine findings of neuroscience, and take full account of the limits to human functioning that accompany dementia, set by structural changes in the brain.

Both ingredients – the ethic and the social psychology – are needed for an approach that is truly person-centred. The ethic alone might provide a motive, but the practical insight and skill to do the task well would be lacking. Many blunders have been committed in the name of kindness and good intent. On the other hand, a social psychology that has no in-built ethic often produces knowledge that lacks vitality and direction; also it tends to remain the property of a non-involved elite, and may serve their academic interest above all else. Only when the ethic and the social psychology are brought together – when values are unashamedly built into our empirical inquiry – does a person-centred approach come into being.

In preparing for this new series of articles we asked a number of people who are very experienced in the field of dementia care, and who are strongly committed to doing it in a person-centred way, to present part of the story of one individual with whom they have been involved. The aim is that they should take some aspect of the care process and tell us in what way it seemed to have good effects. Our briefing to the authors gives them plenty of scope for presenting their material in their own way; but we are asking for attention to detail, and for stories of success (however, we don't mean to imply that care studies published in the *Journal of Dementia Care* past and future do not illustrate person-centred care, and we hope readers will continue to contribute accounts from their experience).

Sharing our experience

It is an important step forward, so I believe, for us to share together our experiences along these lines. We need to leave behind us the old negative images of dementia, and a mind-set that is continually preoccupied with problems. We can find much encouragement and confidence from the things that are going well. The stories have a moral significance, for they show in detail how an ethic of respect for persons becomes a lived reality. They have a social-psychological significance, too, in that they give us glimpses of interpersonal processes that we are only just beginning to understand. Eventually we may even be able to link up these processes with knowledge derived from neuroscience (Damasio 1995). For everything that we describe in social psychological terms has its counterpart in the activities of brains.

In assessing what seems to be the consequence of successful care, a small warning is needed. Whenever a positive outcome occurs (whether in the short or long term), we cannot be sure of the full set of conditions that brought it about. It would be wise to bear in mind at least three main possibilities. The first is that there may be differences between individuals in the type and severity of the neuropathology in their brains; some of these differences may not be detectable by the current methods of neuroscience. The success stories, then, might be occurring mainly with individuals whose functioning is relatively less impaired at a neurological level. Second, there is great variability in the personalities and life histories that individuals bring to their dementia, and hence in their resilience as persons when parts of their brain are undergoing neuropathic change.

Proceed with caution

The third possibility is the one to which we may be most readily drawn. It is that the positive outcome is a direct consequence of the social psychology (or, putting it in other words, the quality of care). It is here that our optimism needs to be tempered with caution.

The truth is that at present there is no way of knowing the relative importance of the three types of factor. We need many more detailed case studies, covering a very wide range of people and conditions. At this stage, however, the following can be said with reasonable confidence. If the quality of care is good, its consequences for the whole population of people with dementia is uncertain; we simply know that there are beneficial effects for some. If, however, the quality of care is poor – permeated by that "malignant social psychology" that I have documented elsewhere (Kitwood 1990) – no individual will be able to withstand its undermining

effects over the course of several years.

The studies that we are going to present, then, are informal and anecdotal. They do not count as research in the true sense, but they are an important preliminary to a kind of inquiry that is very much needed if our knowledge of dementia care is to advance. This would be a careful and systematic investigation of the progress of a large number of individuals through the whole course of their dementing process, right until the point of death, with a large number of variables being taken into account, including key aspects of the care process. Attention would need to be paid to positive changes, both in the long and short term; and ideally, neurological data would be included too. It is only after that kind of research has been done that we will begin to get a sense of the "big picture" of the dementing process, including the kind of long-term outcomes that might reasonably be expected, and in whom. Until then, I suggest that we would do well to suspend all commitment to the so-called stage theories of dementia; these were produced in too much of a hurry, and without any consideration of one of the most crucial of all the variables: the quality of care. (See also Bell & McGregor, 1995). Meanwhile, let's get on with building up our detailed knowledge as best we can.

My guess is that it will be many years yet before all the main pieces of the mosaic of person-centred care are fitted together. There will, no doubt, always be some dark places; some of the anguish and sorrow that surrounds dementia is beyond our power to take away. But each new piece of the mosaic will be a source of fresh strength and confidence; and as it takes its place in the whole pattern, it will shine like a jewel in the light.

References

Bell J, McGregor I (1995) A challenge to stage theories of dementia. In Kitwood T, Benson S (Eds) *The New Culture of Dementia Care*. Hawker Publications, London.

Damasio AR (1995) *Descartes' Error*. Picador, London.

Kitwood T (1990) The dialectics of dementia: with particular reference to Alzheimer's disease. *Ageing and Society* 10 177-196.

Mackie JL (1983) *Ethics*. Penguin, Harmondsworth.

Post SG (1996) *The Moral Challenge of Alzheimer's Disease*. Johns Hopkins, Baltimore.

Through the past to the person

FAITH GIBSON
JO MARLEY
HELEN MᶜVICKER

Relating to a person with dementia who has begun to give up their usual means of communication is a complex and daunting task. In this case study, the authors show how using information from the past, together with detailed observation of the person's present behaviour, helped social workers restore contact, reduce agitation and increase well-being.

Andy and his wife Anna were both in their mid-60s when they were referred to a statutory social services elderly care team, following Andy's diagnosis of Alzheimer's disease by a psychogeriatrician.

Both were born in Belfast and had grown up in the same neighbourhood. They were childhood sweethearts and had married when Anna was 16. Andy was at that time a merchant seaman, but he sought a shore job to be near his wife. He was employed in the Belfast gas works for the rest of his working life except for a short period when the whole family moved to Australia. Andy and Anna had three children, two daughters and a son who all married and set up home in the Belfast area.

Throughout his life Andy had been a quiet, placid and sociable man who enjoyed a joke and a chat, and loved to play his guitar. Anna, on the other hand, was a real character – the life and soul of any gathering. The couple enjoyed a very close relationship which remained throughout the whole course of his deteriorating illness.

Twice-weekly day care had been provided for him, primarily to give his wife time for domestic tasks, shopping and visiting her daughters and son who lived in the neighbourhood. But Andy rapidly deteriorated. His initial Cape Orientation score of 10/12 had changed to 3/12 with accompanying bizarre behaviour by the end of the first year following referral, and he died within the next subsequent year.

When first referred, Andy was a sociable, jovial man who liked to laugh a lot and talk to people. As he deteriorated, he stopped talking, to his wife, other family members and the social worker. At first, although his short-term memory was impaired, he nevertheless talked freely, recounted stories, told jokes and joined in conversation. But over the course of the one year he virtually stopped talking to anyone and had withdrawn into a private world which excluded even his devoted wife of nearly 50 years. She became increasingly distressed by his perpetual silence.

Identifying a pattern

It began to dawn on his social worker, Helen McVicker, that most of what she knew about Andy, she had learned second-hand from others. She rarely asked (or expected) Andy to speak for himself. She became convinced that something more was needed to prevent Andy being abandoned to his encroaching silent, isolated world. Andy's wife also agreed that between them, something must be done, and she willingly agreed to compile a comprehensive diary based on careful observation of her husband's behaviour over several days. Among other things, she charted his periods of restlessness, agitation and unhappiness which for the first time were identified as having a regular pattern. They consistently occurred in the early afternoon after lunch, preceded by a more settled period in the late morning.

In parallel with this detailed observation which concentrated on present behaviour, the social worker began to compile a systematic chronological life history. This process was greatly helped by a well ordered collection of family photographs which chronicled Andy's life in childhood, courtship, marriage, the navy, Australia, employment in the gas works, family events, hobbies – including a love of classical guitar music – holidays and significant people in his life, such as his Aunt Rosie. This information was methodically gathered over a number of weeks by means of carefully planned, non-directive interviews with Andy's wife, who was only too glad to make a positive contribution to her husband's care.

This vivid information then provided the triggers for reminiscence work with Andy and for efforts designed to decrease his early afternoon agitated restlessness by playing him guitar music cassettes. During this time he would lie back in his favourite chair, close his eyes and listen to music for an hour or more. Agitation and anxiety were replaced by relaxation and enjoyment.

Pleasure in recognition

The photographs were also used in the day centre to engage Andy in recognition, recall and conversation about key people and past events. Even when Andy was not able to give names to people or places he clearly indicated his recognition of them and pleasure in being shown the pictures.

When looking with Helen at photographs of a holiday in Canada, Andy recounted an incident at Niagara Falls. Almost automatically Helen interpreted this story as fabrication, a consequence of dementia, but his wife subsequently confirmed the details of the event, accurately recounted by Andy.

The knowledge of this man's life and interests was used to initiate conversation and to locate it within familiar territory. The risk of setting him up for failure was greatly reduced because he was not being confronted with strange general questions unrelated to his own familiar past experience. Helen learned to believe rather than disbelieve the things Andy talked about. In numerous, subtle ways, the fear of being found out or found wanting was reduced and he no longer needed to play safe by retreating into silence.

When Andy died, Anna donated his brain to the Northern Ireland Alzheimer's research brain bank.

She made a number of television appearances and broadcasts to encourage other people to do the same. She became the backbone of a local carer's support group and worked tirelessly to support new carers in similar situations to her own, before her sudden, unexpected death only a few months after her husband.

Contact restored

Andy's deterioration was not miraculously halted by this combination of careful observation and use of his own life history, but his last years were less isolated and his affectionate relationship with his wife continued until his death. To some extent at least, this work succeeded in re-engaging Andy with his wife and his social worker. They were both persuaded that precise and careful observation and detailed life history information together did provide creative ways for helping Andy remain in contact with them, despite his encroaching illness.

Highly sensitive, specifically focused, person-centred work challenges the widely held view that people with dementia become dramatically changed personalities. Such a view all too readily excuses care staff from the effort of understanding what additional threats to well-being, and to personhood, the present care environment – and their own thoughtless behaviour, even if well intentioned – may pose to people with dementia.

2 | Back into the swing of her sociable life

TRACY PETRE

In sheltered housing there is a danger that tenants with advancing dementia will be excluded from social events by other residents. Tracy Petre describes how discovering the unique personality behind a woman's "problem behaviour" led to ways of reducing her frustration, which allowed her to join in the fun again.

Bessy was a woman with advanced dementia, who lived in the sheltered housing scheme Flower Court for several years. Janet, the Warden, summed up her life there: "She had a sparkle. She was very happy here." This is Bessy's story, based on my meetings with her and her daughter, and my conversations with Janet.

High level of well-being

When Bessy moved into Flower Court from a village a few miles away, she was already showing early signs of memory problems that were obvious to her close family. Her daughter lived near the scheme and had applied for a flat for her mother so that she could give her extra help.

Two years later, when I first met Bessy, her dementia had increased considerably: she had no conception of where she was living and made little conversation. Her daughter commented, "You can't have a proper conversation with her, because she doesn't understand anything."

However, Bessy appeared to have a very high level of well-being compared to many other people with dementia I had met. During my visit to her flat she made no real conversation but constantly laughed and made happy fragmented comments. This impression was confirmed by the warden. According to her reports, Bessy always showed a considerable amount of humour, frequently initiated social contact with others and was usually relaxed.

Bit by bit I pieced together clues as to what might have been preserving this high level of well-being. Two factors seemed most important: a strong attachment bond with the warden; plus knowledge of Bessy's previous preferences and habits being used as a base for "problem" solving.

"Problems"

When Bessy first moved into the scheme, the situation was not as happy as I found it two years later. During her first few months in Flower Court she had often been aggressive, and indeed physically violent, towards people who came into conflict with her. For example, she always refused to be undressed for bed and if anyone tried to help her do so she would hit out.

This was a problem for all involved. Her daughter was trying to help but being constantly attacked. Her neighbours were afraid of the aggressive outbursts and so tended to avoid Bessy, which severely restricted her social life.

In addition, a problem of a different kind was occurring. At a similar time every day Bessy would attempt to leave the scheme and search for a bus back to the village where she had previously lived. In sheltered housing, tenants tend to be active enough to come and go as they please and there are no care staff to look out for people. Therefore as Bessy's dementia developed it was a growing concern that she would be lost and/or injured if this behaviour continued.

"Solutions"

Luckily for Bessy, she and Janet the warden had "immediately hit it off", as Janet told me. The two women had "clicked" on their first meeting and over time became strongly bonded to one another. A number of behaviours on Bessy's part confirmed her attachment. For example, she had learnt Janet's name straight away and always used it – "to my surprise," said Janet. If Bessy hurt herself she would search out Janet to help her. On one such occasion she fell and badly hurt her knee and yet still managed to walk to Janet's office, saying to her, "save me".

Because of this strong attachment, Janet was committed to exploring possibilities to lessen Bessy's afternoon disappearances, her aggression and consequent stigmatisation by other tenants. So she arranged to discuss the situation with Bessy's daughter.

What emerged from their conversation was a rich picture of Bessy's previous life. Before her husband had died, the couple had spent their life as publicans. Apparently Bessy had been extremely extrovert and outgoing – she loved company, jokes, dressing up for work and having a firm routine to her life. Obviously this lifestyle also meant that

Bessy needed to be able to protect herself when threatened, even if this was by just appearing aggressive.

Janet had used this personal information to form a few ideas of ways in which she might lessen Bessy's problems. The main initial dilemma was that Bessy refused to undress for bed, becoming aggressive if pushed. Some creative thinking around Bessy's previous love of dressing up eased the situation. The warden allowed Bessy to sleep in the clothes she had worn during the day. The next morning when the home help would visit Bessy, she would get out lots of outfits and comment, "It's like C&A in here, let's try on some clothes." Bessy would then happily try on different things until she was in a new, clean outfit each day.

Turning her attention to Bessy's increasingly dangerous wandering and searching, Janet thought of the boredom she must now be experiencing after such a busy and routine-filled life. As a start to encouraging a new routine, Janet began to take Bessy with her when she took and picked up her children from school. This gave a very regular format to her day. At exactly the same time each morning and afternoon Bessy would go on what she called "an outing", meeting other people as she went, which encouraged her sociable nature.

Following the onset of this routine, and new way of approaching her "difficult behaviours", the warden commented that "Bessy's aggression died down a lot". Little by little, as her frustration and aggression dissolved, her previous outgoing personality returned. Other tenants found that Bessy could be very jovial and a lot of fun to be with.

Joining in the party

With a little encouragement, tenants accepted that Bessy would come to some social events in the communal lounge, and a few would pick her up from her flat. Bessy "had a wonderful time", according to Janet, at these social events. She loved to sing and when tenants walked her back to her flat they would have to sing with her all the way.

Thus the scheme had arrived at the situation I found when I first met Bessy. Bessy was happy and relaxed, strongly attached to Janet. Her initial aggression had lessened considerably without the use of medication. Other tenants had grown to like Bessy and actively helped her to join in events.

Before my most recent visit to Flower Court, Bessy had a serious fall and was admitted to local hospital casualty and subsequently to a geriatric ward. Three weeks later she died while still in hospital.

Until the end of her time in Flower Court, Bessy had remained closely bonded to Janet and well liked by other tenants. On the day of her funeral half of the tenants of the scheme attended and paid their respects – an indication of how well thought of Bessy had been.

Conclusion

This study shows clearly how person-centred care can make a crucial difference to the life of someone with dementia. Bessy had formed a close attachment and friendship with Janet. The alleviation of her initially aggressive reaction to dementia had brought with it renewed sociability and friendships. Although dementia had brought with it many losses for Bessy, something new and valuable was gained.

3 | Amos: a self lost and found

MARGARET ANNE TIBBS

The lack of culturally sensitive services for people from ethnic minorities can literally be deadly – it nearly was for Amos Jackson. Margaret Anne Tibbs describes the life of this Jamaican "grandfather figure" who came to the UK in the 1960s and the lessons it taught her.

This is the story of Amos Jackson. He was born and grew up in Jamaica – a Maroon, descended from the earliest inhabitants of the island. He worked on banana plantations and was also a lay preacher. Like many other people from the Caribbean islands, he came to Bedford to work in the local brickworks in the 1960s.

Later he met and fell in love with Hesther, with whom he had two daughters. Hesther had been married before and had children of her own. For many years they lived together in her house. Sadly, differences developed between them, and although Amos remained steadfastly devoted to her, he moved out to live on his own.

Then Hesther became increasingly frail. She had severe arthritis and diabetes. After she had a slight stroke it was arranged by the family that Amos should move back into the house to look after her. For a time the arrangement worked very well. Hesther would organise the household from her armchair, doing the thinking and planning for both of them, and Amos would be her hands and feet, carrying out her instructions. With help from home carers provided by social services they were able to live as an independent unit.

But then Amos began to forget things. He seemed unable to carry out Hesther's instructions, and became subject to apparently irrational outbursts of anger. Eventually a diagnosis of multi-infarct dementia was made in 1991. By the end of 1992 he could no longer honour his part of the bargain. The family increased their support, but despite this, every week seemed to bring a fresh crisis.

Then Hesther had another stroke and was admitted to the general hospital. The family had a real emergency on their hands because it was clear to everyone that Amos could not now be left safely on his own at home. It was arranged that he should stay with his daughter for a few days. Unfortunately she was not experienced in looking after someone with dementia. Something happened – I was never able to ascertain exactly what, but Amos had one of his outbursts of aggression – a knife was involved. The GP was called and Amos was admitted to the local psychiatric hospital as an informal patient for a three-week assessment. Initially the family were relieved.

Downhill slide

From this point on it was downhill all the way for Amos. He had four great disadvantages. He was a man. He was a big man. He was a big black man. And he had a history of aggression. Towards the end of three weeks his case was discussed in a multi-disciplinary meeting. By that time this man, who before admission had been out and about in the town he knew well and helping with household chores, was in a sorry state.

This man who had been regarded by his community and family as a rather eccentric grandfather figure had become doubly incontinent, could hardly walk and rarely spoke except when he became angry and abusive. It was decided on this evidence that he was too ill to be discharged home. As the weeks turned into months, he lost weight, ceased to speak and presented all the signs of a man in the later stages of dementia. It was presumed by the medical staff that he had suffered another major infarct and that he would need 24-hour care – probably in a psychiatric hospital – for the rest of his life.

Hesther's daughter Delores, who was in effect Amos's main carer, was becoming increasingly desperate as Amos sank further and further into decline. She felt quite powerless. All her requests to have him discharged home were disregarded even though he had been admitted as an informal patient. From the evidence available to the medical staff, it did indeed seem by this stage that Amos was terminally ill. He had stopped eating or speaking and he no longer even became angry.

Eventually a friend of Delores who was also from the Caribbean came to work in the local social services department and she showed Delores how to make a formal complaint in writing, and to request that care in the community for Amos should at least be tried.

Another case conference was called and it was

agreed that Amos could go home on a trial basis on condition that 24-hour care was provided for him and that the case was supervised by the specialist social worker for dementia – me. Therefore, in July 1992, five months after his admission to hospital, Amos went home. I have tried to imagine what life must have been like for Amos in the psychiatric hospital, where he was the only Caribbean patient in a large ward (although there was a young care assistant who was also of African descent), being offered strange tasting food, where he often could neither understand, nor be understood, because he spoke in a strong Jamaican dialect. I think he just gave up. I think he was indeed at death's door – but not because of his dementia.

Before he went home a rota of carers was set up to provide 24-hour supervision and care, for both himself and Hesther who had been discharged from hospital and was still living in the house. As the social worker, I spent some time educating the carers about the nature of multi-infarct dementia and working out strategies for dealing with Amos's behaviour with them. The linchpin of the care package was Milly, who came every day with her little boy Joshua, a lively six-year-old, to look after the two old people. She could only earn a limited amount of money without losing her benefits, and other members of the care team were in the same position. It therefore suited them to work for a rate of pay which was well below that charged by private care agencies.

Perversely, this had worked against them in the previous assessment because they were perceived as being "benefit scroungers". What was not appreciated was that they also did it because they all belonged to the Jamaican community and the same Pentecostal church. They felt it to be their Christian duty and they genuinely cared for Amos. Delores filled in the gaps in the rota. Social services continued to provide home carers to look after Hesther's needs.

Back to his old self

Within a month of returning home Amos was back to his old self. It seemed like a miracle that this could be the same man I had seen in the hospital. He was often able to hold a lucid conversation. The family took him to church and out on the bus to town. He enjoyed walking with an escort to the shops. A deeply religious man, he would spend hours listening to his gospel tapes or to a portion of scripture being read to him.

It was Milly who suggested to me that the aggressive episodes might be caused by arthritic pain in his neck and shoulders. Sometimes Amos

thought he was in Jamaica and would insist that he had to go out to the yard to pick bananas. But the family were tolerant of these forays into his past. They knew where he was coming from, in every sense.

Sadly, his beloved Hesther had another stroke and died about seven months later. Delores took him to see her body and he remembered from that time on that she was dead. He would stand at the window as it grew dark and talk about her. The family decided to continue to care for Amos in Hesther's house.

The care package still worked well to support him after her death for several more months. Eventually, however, Hesther's house was needed for another family member, and Milly's circumstances also changed which meant that she could no longer give as much time as she had to the care of Amos. The time arrived when he had to move into a residential home.

Delores looked at several and eventually chose one which suited him really well. As soon as Amos saw his bedroom he made it clear that he felt at home there. Delores told me how he stood at the window and waved goodbye to her when she left him there, smiling happily. The family visit often. Whenever Amos becomes agitated, which he still does, the staff take him to his room and turn on his gospel tapes. They leave him alone in peace, keeping him under discreet observation. They learned from Delores that this is the best way to manage these episodes.

If the weather permits they take him out to the enclosed garden where he can sit on his own. He needs to have his own space and the staff understand this. His arthritic pain is now properly controlled for the first time.

I saw him last three months ago, and he honestly seemed little different from the man I had seen in his own home a year before. He did however seem totally different from the wreck of a man I had seen in the psychiatric hospital – a man who had literally and metaphorically turned his face to the wall.

The case taught me so much. How a system designed to care for people can actually abuse them. How the lack of culturally sensitive services for people from ethnic minorities can be deadly – as it nearly was in this case. How the people who really knew what Amos needed were those closest to him – his family; and yet how totally without power this family was until Delores' friend acted as their advocate.

Until we learn to focus on the person – the whole person, the whole life – our well-meant efforts to help will never be enough. In this case, fortunately, the system did manage to listen before it was too late, and Amos is alive and well to prove it.

4 | Driven by fear to defend his secure world

GRAHAM STOKES

Mr D's tormented, disturbing behaviour was incomprehensible to those around him. Understanding its roots could not give him the peace of mind he had never possessed, but it brought tolerance and greatly lessened his wife's distress, writes Graham Stokes.

I first became acquainted with Mr D when his wife informally sought my services at a neighbourhood resource centre. She reported months of increasing worry as her husband became ever more absent-minded and argumentative. His lapses of memory were puzzling, and at times irritating, but of greater concern was his odd behaviour. He would complain, for example, that it was not possible to open the front door if he had a newspaper in one hand and a briefcase in the other, and hesitated when confronted with the familiar task of crossing the road.

What brought matters to a head, however, was the christening of their first grandchild. Having attended the ceremony and returned to their daughter's for a celebratory lunch, Mr D could not be found. Eventually he was seen sitting patiently outside in their car. Walking toward the vehicle Mrs D recalled thinking her husband was being antisocial and listening to the radio – an action consistent with the personality of an insular man, yet "surely not at the christening of his own grandchild".

She was correct. Mrs D knew her husband well enough to know he would never be so insensitive, but the knowledge did not prepare her for what she was about to experience. He demanded to go home, saying that to stay any longer would mean dinner being late. At first staggered and disbelieving, and then exasperated, she pleaded for her husband to be sensible.

But within his tortured world he was already being so. It was not that he was unable to recall the purpose of their visit; his determined protestations to return home reflected a desperate need to be safe, to feel secure and emotionally comfortable. His home was a sanctuary offering routine and predictability. He knew what was expected of him, where everything was in its place, and there was a place for everything. He did not wish to go into an unfamiliar house and sit next to people whose names he should know but could not remember; he did not wish to suffer the embarrassment of not knowing what to do next; nor did he want to see again that expression on a person's face that betrayed the fact he was now repeating himself.

The diagnosis

Over the following months discreet investigations and observation by myself and the family doctor (for Mr D would not acknowledge there was a problem) yielded a probable diagnosis of Alzheimer's disease. He was 58 years old.

As Mr D progressively deteriorated he became profoundly forgetful of new or recent events. He retired from work and sold his group of small corner supermarkets. Disoriented and dependent, he exacted a heavy toll on his wife's welfare. She described her husband as a "born worrier" and unsurprisingly his behaviour became increasingly agitated.

Domiciliary support and respite care were offered by social services, but refused. Mrs D felt that her husband would not accept the presence of strangers within his domain, nor would he adjust to the mysterious unknown world of care. Her concerns were confirmed by the sole attempt to provide day care. Mr D became so anxious he attempted to climb out of a window rather than stay in the company of people he did not know, within a building he did not recognise.

The challenge

For Mrs D, and without doubt Mr D (who was one of the most tormented people with dementia I have ever met) there was to be a distressing turn of events. A set of behaviours appeared that were to earn him the name Rock Man, and all but destroy the health of his devoted wife. These behaviours were dismissed by most professionals involved as challenging, difficult and symptomatic of the presumed cerebral pathology.

Mr D was driven, day after day, to collect rocks and large stones from his gardens and store them in neat piles in his garage. From early morning to the end of the day, he would work in the garden. Collecting his wheelbarrow and spade he would walk to a flower-bed and systematically destroy it. Flowers, shrubs and small trees were pulled out or hacked down.

He would then shovel as much soil as he could into the wheelbarrow, and wheel his barrow onto the lawn where he would empty the contents. Separating the soil from the rocks and stones, he would wheel the latter to his garage. Returning to the garden he would gather up as much soil as his judgement would allow and deposit it onto the flower bed.

As the weeks passed he destroyed his gardens. His wife pleaded to no avail. Efforts to stop him would be met with anger and resistance. At times his hands would be bloodied and bruised, but he would not, could not stop. At the end of the day he would pace the house, ultimately to fall into an exhausted sleep.

For no identifiable reason Mr D would occasionally vary his behaviour. Instead of wheeling his barrow onto the lawn, he would bring it into the house and empty its contents onto the carpet. The hall and lounge carpets became damp, dirty and home to a large number of bugs.

Eventually, his behaviour escalated to the point whereby Mrs D not only struggled with her own bitterness and resentment ("Why me, why us?", "Why is he doing this to me?"), but with the fury of her neighbours, for Mr D would now walk into the street to accost passers-by. His speech was now indistinct and predominantly incoherent. Yet he was clearly expressing concerns and worry. On occasions he would take it upon himself to go into neighbours' gardens armed with his barrow and spade, and attempt to – well, what? What were his intentions?

For most people who knew him, motivation was an irrelevant consideration. His behaviour was regarded as devoid of meaning, being seen as conduct typical of a dementia sufferer who could never be labelled "pleasantly confused".

Therapeutic suggestions hinged on a need to contain the problem. Sedation was regularly advised, as was removal to a secure living arrangement elsewhere. His wife, however, would not "let go", nor did she wish to lose her husband to a world of withdrawn disengagement, even though his presence was a constant reminder of his apparent absence rather than his existence. For Mrs D this was a time of helplessness and despair. To be told her husband's behaviour was because he had dementia offered neither solace or solution.

The person acknowledged

Mr D's conduct was, however, not meaningless. Patient observation of his behaviour, entering into communication that focused on non-verbal signals, and giving his wife the opportunity to talk at length about her husband, resulted in an understanding of who her husband was and who he remained. His perplexing behaviour resonated meaning, but his deconstructed behavioural patterns served to obscure his psychology rather than providing a gateway to his inner world of need and feeling.

It was not difficult to establish the distressed and driven nature of his destructive conduct. Yet why were rocks and stones of such significance? Why was there a need to hide them away? Talking to his wife revealed a man who had, as the years passed, become increasingly concerned about personal safety and the security of their home. The latter point was uncovered when Mrs D expressed bewilderment that this man who valued his home to the extent that he had placed ornamental wrought iron bars over insecure windows was determined to destroy his property. This line of conversation exposed an enduring psychological need being acted out through a deed rooted in personal history.

Mr D had been dedicated to the management of his stores, working long hours and most days, yet he was also a caring, although remote, husband and father. Throughout his life, Mr D had been tormented by worries and anxieties, most of which were inconsequential. Possibly as a means of gaining both security and relief he developed an obsessional personality, becoming preoccupied with detail and punctuality.

His rigid adherence to a predictable lifestyle was unfortunately to lead to a personal disaster. On a Friday evening 15 years earlier he had closed one of his shops and, as was his custom, was leaving the store to bank the day's takings. As he was closing the door, three youths ran across the road to snatch the money bag. He saw them coming and was able to get back into the shop and slam the door shut.

As they hammered on the door, he ran through the store to an office at the rear of the shop from where he could telephone the police. Not prepared to give up, the youths ran to a builder's skip a few yards away, removed pieces of masonry and threw it through the window of the shop.

They climbed through the shattered window and ran through the store to where Mr D was trapped in an office, behind a door that could not be locked. This anxious and insecure man must have been consumed with dread and foreboding. Fortunately, for reasons which never became clear, the youths hesitated, turned on their heels and ran off empty-handed.

Fifteen years on, Mr D continued to wrestle with his enduring need to be safe, but his strategy for fulfilment was now contaminated by the historical entering the "here and now" as if it was painful reality. His conviction was that his home, his secure world, would be attacked in the same way his shop had been. His motivation was to protect himself and his wife from such hazards. The emotions associated with the attempted robbery were no longer tempered by the passage of time but were felt with the force of the original moment, and they generated a powerful motive for action.

Mr D's devastated capacity to reason prevented him from appreciating that people rarely, if ever, attack your home with rocks and stones from your garden. The point of significance is, however, that a person with dementia will select a manner of behaving which is appropriate to them in light of how they interpret their experiences; an interpretation that is subjective, not objective.

Intervention and outcome

There was no successful resolution in terms of giving Mr D what he had never possessed – peace of mind. However, understanding does not only help find solutions, but it can generate tolerance, as the behaviour loses its mystery. With tolerance comes the potential to cope, even with situations that are basically unchanged.

This was the outcome for this couple. Once the probable roots of her husband's behaviour were exposed Mrs D became better equipped to cope. She was no longer terrorised by a belief that he was deliberately acting to hurt or spite, nor was she condemned to live with a person whom she had felt was no longer the man she had once known and loved, despite the physical evidence to the contrary.

Mrs D and her husband went to his family's home in Ireland for a two-week break, during which time their sons arranged for the gardens to be tidied and a secure gate to be placed at the end of the drive. The downstairs carpets were replaced and I advised Mrs D on her return to make sure that when her husband went into the garden both the front and back doors were locked.

The most damaging consequences of his conduct thus prevented, Mr D was able to continue his driven behaviour without interference. He was no longer confronted with demands to stop. The progressive aphasia that was taking away his speech and comprehension prevented verbal acknowledgement of his fears. However, reassuring him by touch and tone of voice that his actions were OK; and even sometimes, when he was seen to be struggling, colluding with his efforts to collect rocks, combined to bring him temporary relief. It was a transient sense of well-being, lasting no longer than the duration of his memory span (how long?). Yet such supportive gestures are not diminished by their fleeting benefits. To bring moments of comfort and reassurance to a person lost in a mysterious and threatening world is a valued objective, never to be underestimated.

Mrs D also derived comfort from the knowledge that as the dementia progressed his failing capacity to recall would lead to a loss of the distressing memory. He would no longer be motivated to hide away rocks and stones, and thus the strain of caring would be greatly diminished. This was how the story unfolded. During the remaining months of destructive behaviour Mrs D was a more effective and confident supporter. As time passed her husband slowly became less preoccupied with the significance of collecting rocks. His behaviour acquired the characteristic of a habit from which he was more easily discouraged. Mrs D continued to care for her husband at home as he became grossly dependent. Eventually he was admitted to hospital with a serious chest infection. Mr D failed to recover and died 17 days later. He was 63.

5 | Perfect manners demand a first-class service

DAPHNE WALLACE

A stickler for correctness and punctuality, George resents a casual approach but responds well when addressed as if by the deferential staff of a hotel or club offering him first-class service! Daphne Wallace describes how an understanding of George's personality has influenced his care.

George and his wife lived in a pleasant bungalow in a quiet cul-de-sac. In their early 70s with a grown-up family, she was content to look after the house while George, retired from his own business, played golf with his many friends.

George had always been very meticulous and precise. He controlled the finances in the household and was the main instigator of the routine of their lives. He was the one who often organised the groups to go for a game of golf. Throughout his life he has been precise and a stickler for "correctness".

In the same way that he organised his life, he organised his possessions. He was always impeccably dressed and had drawers filled with rows of socks, shirts, etc, which were meticulously arranged and had to be kept absolutely tidy at all times. Ties, socks and shirts were always painstakingly matched and coordinated.

One day when George woke up his wife could not follow his conversation. Over the next week or so the situation did not improve – in fact it got worse. Eventually, he was admitted to the local hospital for investigations. In the general medical ward he did not settle; he was unaware that he was in hospital or that the people around him were nurses and fellow patients; in fact he thought he was in a club. He repeatedly tried to leave, insisting that he was going home with his wife.

Polite but resentful

When I was asked to see him he was extremely resentful that a mere woman was asking him what he saw as irrelevant questions, although he was polite when actually speaking to me. As he had no realisation that he was in hospital (despite being told so repeatedly) it was impossible to obtain agreement to transfer to a psychiatric unit for assessment. He was therefore admitted under the Mental Health Act.

In the assessment ward he repeatedly tried to leave – attempting to take with him the golf party he had assembled. (There were at least two other golfers in the ward, one of whom was a member of the same club.) By this time he was convinced that he was in a club or hotel and that he had a car parked outside. On occasions when he got out he tried to get into the parked cars outside to see if they were his. At times he became aggressive when he had to be brought back to the ward; a small dose of haloperidol, however, seemed to limit this hostile response.

Smart and persuasive

Unfortunately he remained determined to leave and realised that the digital lock was the only thing keeping him in. He retained his smart appearance, was often mistaken for a visitor, and on occasion persuaded someone to open the door for him. As a result he had to have his Mental Health Act order extended, and as yet it has not been possible to change this although as he becomes more settled I hope that it will soon. The diagnosis reached is that he is suffering from a moderate degree of dementia, almost certainly of vascular, multi-infarct type.

Both George and his wife now live in the hospital. His wife is a patient on our assessment ward with rapidly progressing dementia, and George lives in our continuing care ward.

For much of the time he is quite settled and cooperative. He knows that the board on the wall tells him where he is, and reads out the hospital name, but he still talks as if he is in a hotel, commenting on how busy the restaurant is or asking if I've had my lunch there. He still tries to leave at every opportunity, though with the most polite of manners. If the door to the garden is open he loves to go out but has to be watched as, given half a chance, he will climb the fence.

Recently he has on a couple of occasions got out of the ward but come back of his own accord. I hope that this means we will soon be able to remove all restrictions.

Meticulous about time-keeping

How has our knowledge of his personality affected the way we care for him? Despite his disorientation in place and appalling short-term memory he is meticulous about time. It is no good distracting him with, "in a minute George", or "I'll be finished in five minutes". He returns on the dot of the appropriate time suggested and is irritated that you have not kept the appointment.

He has always been an active man and he loves to walk. At every opportunity staff, especially male staff to whom he relates much better, take him for a walk. Sometimes they just take him with them if they have to go elsewhere in the hospital or when staffing allows they take him for a walk in the grounds.

His manners and appearance remain impeccable and he would resent being spoken to in a careless way. Mealtimes are important and the table has to be correctly laid: after all, he believes he is in a club or hotel and he expects first-class service! As he has got to know the staff he is much more cooperative – though only when spoken to as if by deferential staff in a hotel. At times he is doubtful about taking his medication but is pleased to accept it if told that it has been sent specially for him by the management.

When he stands at the ward door hoping to get out, it is possible to ask him politely to go in the opposite direction to help someone. If he was told "You can't go out there", he would become resentful.

Relationships

His family find that it is possible to take him out for the day as long as they do not go back to his own house. At present he recognises his family but when they are not there he may think another patient is his wife – much to the fury of the husband of one when he visits.

When his own wife visits he greets her by name but soon tires and goes off to another part of the ward. She becomes very upset by this and has recently stated that she does not want to visit. She even told my ward doctor that he was dead.

He has not formed an attachment to any particular person though he seems to relate particularly well to his key worker – a male nurse whom he addresses by name.

Helping him feel at home

It is very important to help him to maintain his smart appearance and he still can be mistaken for a visitor unless one tries to have a conversation. Certain things seem to help him to feel at home. He loves time to talk to people and always enjoys his newspaper. He watches sport on TV, especially golf, which seems to hold his attention well.

I still hope that he will become settled enough to become an informal patient, and if that happens he will not need to be in hospital. Meanwhile, we try very hard to maintain the kind of ordered and friendly routine that he is used to. We do try to explain that he is in a hospital but we also try to meet his demands which would be more appropriate in a hotel.

We are now able to carry out a gradual reduction in medication without return to his previous irritable behaviour. I am sure this is largely because of the greater understanding we now have of him as a person.

6 Hiding in the depths of distress

JOAN COSTELLO

How do you begin to give person-centred care when distress has forced that person into hiding deep within herself? Separation from her husband Ted pushed Vera more quickly and more deeply into her isolation. With hindsight, her care team realised that what was really needed was a commitment to help the couple restore their life together.

Vera Browning came to Westbury after she had been found by the police wandering on the motorway in icy cold weather, dressed only in her nightdress and bare feet. To make matters worse, her husband Ted had slipped on the ice and been taken to casualty that day. These events were the final straw, but problems had been building up for some time. She frequently got lost and had been pulling out plants in her neighbour's garden, saying she was searching for something. Both Ted and the warden of their sheltered housing had reluctantly decided they couldn't cope any longer.

That afternoon I went to visit her in the hospital day room. I had met her briefly three weeks previously, and it was a shock to see how she was changed. She sat in the corner, her eyes closed, not in sleep but to block out thoughts of where she was and how she came to be there.

I asked the nurse to leave us for a while, waited for a moment or two and then said, "May I sit with you, Mrs Browning?" Her eyes opened momentarily: "You do what you like, dear."

I used the moment of drawing up a chair to think "What do I do next?" but Vera herself made the next move.

"Are you a doctor?" she asked. "What are they going to do with me?"

"No, I'm not a doctor, but I think both of us together can sort things out."

"Where's Ted?" she asked. "Why doesn't he come?"

I told her Ted had fallen on the ice, that I had been to see him in hospital, that he had hurt his leg and wasn't able to walk just yet. I said I knew she had been through a very frightening time. I tried hard to feel her pain, her isolation, her inability to understand what was happening and what had happened to her world. I touched her arm gently, all the time afraid she might close her eyes and shut me out again.

"Where is Ted? Why don't they let me see him?" were the only words she said, over and over again.

I felt very inadequate in this situation. All I could do was to acknowledge her loneliness and fear: "It must be very lonely for you without Ted. Can I share your company for a little while? Then I will go to see Ted again."

She nodded in assent and made no move to send me away, so for some time we sat together. No words were said but I felt that Vera was more at peace. When I felt that it was time to leave and stood up to go she said: "Do you know where Ted lives?" I felt then that I had broken a little of the shell of her imposed isolation.

Deep loneliness

Transition from home to hospital, and subsequently to residential care, is in itself a terrible burden for someone with dementia to carry. Vera had to make this transition without much of the family support which had always been there for her. This had left her in a totally submissive state, holding deep within herself the loneliness and the loss of the world she had known. Her mind blocked out the frightening events now thrust upon her.

In hospital Vera had been prescribed a neuroleptic drug to ease her distress. This helped temporarily each time it was given, but then her troubles recurred with greater devastation. Now Vera found herself in a state of utter bewilderment. She had overwhelming problems but she no longer had a mind which was able to produce solutions acceptable to the world she saw around her. Panic had given way to hiding somewhere deep within herself.

But what of Ted? All the loss, the loneliness and feelings of guilt had descended on him. "What is happening to Vera? What can I do?" he asked over and over again. This was of as much concern to me as Vera herself. We would need all his support and he was in no condition to provide it.

Vera's arrival at Westbury presented no special problems. Marilyn, Vera's daughter, had brought her own two children with her in the car, which turned out to be a great help. Their chatter and attention to their Granny had given the journey a happy atmosphere and eased the tension of arrival.

It was after their departure that Vera became disturbed. She called for Ted and walked around incessantly, though a little unsteadily due to the effects of her medication. We explained again and again that Ted was in the hospital with a broken leg and that it would be a few days before he could visit her.

By evening time her fears and anxieties had deepened. She was now convinced that Ted had died: "Where is he? Why doesn't he come? He must be dead." The words were poured out in desperation. Eileen, her key worker, decided eventually to try the hospital. If Ted was still awake, would it be possible to get a mobile phone to him? Minutes later Vera and Ted spoke to each other for the first time since their recent tragedies. "Ted, Ted," was all she was able to say, but she clutched the phone to herself long after the call was over. Eileen told her gently, "Ted has gone to sleep now", and sat with her until she too dropped off to sleep in the chair, as she had resisted all persuasion to get into bed.

The daily contact with Ted became a vital part of the immediate care plan.

Unresponsive?

During those early days at Westbury Vera would not respond to anyone, either staff or other residents. She had withdrawn into herself but was unable to draw any comfort or reassurance from her own thoughts.

What we did not appreciate was that this was Vera's only way of coping with her situation. We saw it as part of her dementia, together with adverse parts of her personality. Staff would comment that she was uncooperative and that she would refuse her food, even spitting it out on occasions.

Vera's key worker, Eileen, became despondent, feeling that she had failed because she was getting no response. This was particularly disappointing after her success with the telephone call.

The staff felt it would be good for Vera to come into the lounge more often to relieve her loneliness. They took her to the "Singalong" and tried to get her involved in other activities. Vera's response was to leave and wander around until she found some corner in which to sit or stand by herself. Eileen tried taking her out to the shops, but her reaction was completely negative. The pattern of being labelled as unresponsive was taking shape. Vera's continual calling "Where is Ted?" was seen as a sign of distress.

Despite our requests to reduce or discontinue the prescribed Melleril 25mg, three times a day, her GP and CPN both felt it important to continue, to relieve this anxiety and distress.

Marilyn, Vera's daughter, tried hard at first but visits became progressively shorter. Vera didn't always recognise her, and Marilyn found her antisocial ways distressing.

Reunion

Eventually, Ted was able to visit Westbury regularly. Post-operative complications had delayed this for some weeks. Now he looked thin and drawn as he hobbled in with a stick.

We had anticipated that Ted's first visit would be an emotional affair, but we were not prepared for the actual event. Vera was almost overcome. "They told me you were dead," she repeated again and again. She clung to him in tears, unable to believe that this really was Ted.

Together with both Vera and Ted, Eileen began to piece together a profile of Vera. Both enjoyed recalling many memories of their early life. They looked at photographs together and laughed. We learned that Vera was an only child, very bright at school. She and Ted had both been brought up in Stepney, London. She was born in 1928; Ted in 1921. We gathered they had been sweethearts from the time Vera had first left school and remained so despite separation during Ted's army service during the war.

There were many differences in their personalities. Vera had a great love of music and ballet. In the early days she had taught dancing. Ted was more into football and darts, but he had always taken Vera to concerts, and when they could afford it, even to the ballet.

Remembered agony

Ted recounted his war stories and told us that at one time he had been listed as "missing, presumed killed", but that in actual fact he had been taken as a prisoner of war. Vera gave quite an amazing response at this point. She told us how she had felt when she was told Ted had been killed: "I cried for days. Then one day they told me he was coming home. We all went to the station to meet him." Vera poured out all her remembered agony.

Now we could understand the depth of Vera's fear and anxiety when Ted was in hospital with his broken leg and she was alone. The reliving of that wartime drama had lifted her distress to unimagined heights. Now we could look at Vera's withdrawal with much greater understanding. It was her way of coping with the awful situation from her past which recurred in a new guise.

Little by little we built up a profile which showed Vera's true self. We saw her now as a shy, quiet person with great inner strength. Ted said many times, "You are my anchor, Vera."

It was clear now that our care plan had to centre

on a shared experience, retaining as much of Ted and Vera's marriage as possible. Getting Ted to Westbury whenever we could was vital, and fortunately we were able to arrange for a volunteer driver to bring him in when he couldn't make it on the bus.

Most days Ted and Vera would sit together on the settee, sometimes chatting, sometimes quiet, just listening to some of their old favourites in music. They enjoyed a meal together, usually in Vera's room. Vera no longer refused to eat. Progressively they put together a more complete life, even having an afternoon nap together. We were prompted to think that what we really needed was a double bed.

The objectives of our care plan were coming together. Vera smiled sometimes and began to display some of her old elegance and grace. We saw her one day showing off some dance steps to another resident. Ted and Vera both knew that they would never recover all of their lost life, but now they would be able to hold together the threads of their relationship. Last week they went to their daughter's for Sunday lunch. Perhaps one day Ted will be able to treat Vera to one of those special days cherished from earlier times. He may even take her to a ballet performance.

Much has been lost from Vera's life. Surrounded as she is by other residents and staff, it is difficult for her to find even a limited part of her former role

as a wife, and this was the one she cherished above all others.

Lessons learned

When we look back now we can see that in those early days at Westbury, we were really compounding Vera's difficulties. Now we see the factors that contributed to her distress, which we couldn't see when it mattered most.

The rapid change of events disempowered Vera. Separation from Ted pushed her more quickly and more deeply into her isolation and that bewildering feeling of no longer being in control of her mind. The high dosage of Melleril had so dulled Vera's senses that although it relieved her anxiety for a brief period its return found her less and less able to cope with distress.

There was our lack of understanding of Vera herself. Now that we have a more complete profile we see clearly how inadequate our first picture was.

We did not fully accept that the care of both people in a partnership must be our responsibility, and that we neglected that to the detriment of both.

Looking back, we see that we merely responded to the crisis in Ted and Vera's lives in the manner which was patterned for us. Maybe in the future we will have gained the confidence and courage to put our resources not into containment, but into the risks of trying to enable couples like Ted and Vera to restore their lives, either at home or in residential care.

7 | Expressing her grief in the only way she knew

ANTHEA INNES
While other staff and residents had reached a point of intolerance, the author could see the warm, sociable lady hidden beneath Mrs G's difficult behaviour. The person-centred approach came too late for her, but her story taught some important lessons.

Mrs G had been a popular and very busy lady. She had many friends, who sent her a total of 140 Christmas cards one year. She had cared for her husband at home when he became ill with Parkinson's disease, while also returning to work to bring in a regular income.

When her husband died she would often go to her son's house to cook dinner for when he and his family returned after work.

Neighbours and friends were always welcome at Mrs G's house, her regular visitors assured me. She had always been friendly to everyone and keen to lend a hand if she was needed. She had got on well with all her neighbours, although latterly she turned on them, accusing them of stealing from her. They couldn't understand why she sometimes made them feel unwelcome when they visited her in the home; she seemed a different person from the one they had known for 60 years.

Mrs G had also turned her back on religion, when previously she had been a regular churchgoer and very active in the local community.

As I got to know her, it seemed to me that she had turned against those who were close to her when she came into the home because she blamed them for the fact that she hadn't been able to continue living in her own home.

I was drawn to Mrs G when I first began working there. She could be warm and friendly one minute, and very cruel and unkind the next; but she was a useful ally when I was setting up activities – she loved to join in. She particularly liked singing and dancing and would often grab me for an impromptu whirl round the room. She would sing as she walked around, telling everyone that she had a lovely voice. She enjoyed baking and would encourage others to come and join in.

She told me she looked forward to me coming in: she obviously liked having something to do. Over the next few months she would often be waiting by the window for me to arrive, and would rush to greet me. On Monday evenings she would tell me that she had got the other ladies to join in a singsong or play with the ball over the weekend when I was off.

She always enjoyed an outing and would be very excited in anticipation of a trip to the theatre or local church show. She would be ready hours before the entertainments organiser arrived.

Getting to know her

She began to tell me more about herself – how she had been quite pretty with bright ginger hair, when she was young. She was concerned that her hair was grey now, that she looked old. Hand massages and manicures were something she greatly enjoyed, and during these one-to-one sessions I discovered much about her. She had lost weight and didn't think her thinner frame became her: she liked to have "a bit of meat on her bones". She blamed her weight loss on the food she was given in the home. If she had been in her own house, she implied, she would have fed herself better.

It became apparent to me early on that she really craved her old life and her old flat. She had "escaped" from the home many times and was missing overnight on one occasion. A new locking system was put on the front door to prevent Mrs G and others leaving the home and forgetting to return. She told me she felt like a prisoner, that she wanted to be at home. I began to understand the reasons for her behaviour.

She shared a room and this was something she detested. She had always had her own space and had lived on her own since her husband died. To be in a double room with only a partition must have gone against the grain. The home's management recognised that Mrs G would like a single room but there wasn't one available. She took to destroying her room-mate's property, hiding clothes, throwing items out the window. All this was an expression of her wish to be at home, on her own.

Staff would often warn me that Mrs G was in a terrible mood, but I would find her to be quite the opposite. She liked to be busy, doing something. However, her amiable days were countered by days when she would begin to participate then decide that throwing a ball was too childish and disrupt the whole game. She liked to help others but would often intervene in what they were doing in a way that was offensive to them. Quizzes were something else she enjoyed, but sometimes she became very disruptive, shouting out answers, swearing and making fun of the other residents.

Mrs G could become very unkind; she was able to pinpoint the weaknesses of other residents and then comment on them, and would often upset certain individuals. Her ability to recognise others' weaknesses led to a general perception that Mrs G knew what she was doing and was behaving in an offensive way deliberately.

Stories friends and relatives told of a quiet, friendly and kind woman didn't match staff experience of working with her. Other residents who were able to understand a bit about dementia threw me very sceptical glances when I tried to explain to them that Mrs G throwing her glass of water instead of the dice when it was her turn at ludo wasn't deliberate; she had genuinely picked up the wrong thing. Mrs G had gone from being a very popular person whose company was sought by others, to being someone who I was often asked to make sure didn't sit by them. Staff and residents were coming to the stage of intolerance, and beyond, trying to understand why Mrs G behaved the way that she did.

The local community psychiatric nurse (CPN) was brought in to talk to staff about working with people with dementia, in particular Mrs G. She had known Mrs G for some years and painted a picture similar to the one I had developed through talking to her friends.

I found the CPN's image of Mrs G to be very enlightening, and other staff too said they had gained insights. However, the reality of working with her was at such odds with what she had been like that the CPN's talk came, I think, too late. Experience and knowledge of Mrs G now took precedence over insights of her in the past.

Problems continued

A few weeks after the CPN's visit staff were still having problems. Some management/prevention strategies were taken on board, such as removing all glasses and cutlery from the dining room where they were kept, as Mrs G repeatedly removed every single item and hid them in her bedroom.

Staff began to keep a record of everything that Mrs G did, in an effort to learn and cope. Yet my experience of Mrs G was still very different from that of other staff. She enjoyed the activities I was there to do, and although there were times when she was disruptive, in the main she was an eager participant. She retained her generous disposition; if she won a prize when playing bingo she would share it round.

I believe Mrs G had become very isolated. She could understand comments that other residents made about her, and she understood all too well when a well-meaning friend told her that her son was selling her flat.

This caused Mrs G great anxiety. She realised if her flat was sold she wouldn't be able to return home. I noticed a great change in her at this point. Her disruptive behaviour escalated. She became a more reluctant participant in activities. One evening she said: "I'm never going to get out of here unless it's in a box, am I?" She understood her situation with great clarity, and spoke like this many times.

I think her disruptive behaviour did have a purpose – to express her unhappiness in the only way she was able. I think she hoped that she would get "thrown out" for being a nuisance. But at the same time I don't think she fully understood her actions; she did like to please people, could be very charming and would often want to help others. I don't believe she meant to make extra work for staff. She was just desperately unhappy.

Attempts were made to try and understand Mrs G, both her behaviours and her personality as a whole. However, a person-centred approach came too late. Perhaps if knowledge of Mrs G as she was before she came into the home and before she developed dementia had been made known early on, a different programme of care would have evolved.

Knowing Mrs G has shaped my approach to the people I work with. Finding out about a person is crucial in understanding why they behave the way they do. Knowledge of the person before they had dementia gives insights into how best to care for that person. In the case of Mrs G, knowledge that she was generous, friendly and very active helped me to understand her and in a way empathise with her situation as she understood it.

Mrs G was taken into hospital after an unfortunate incident one weekend. The details were hazily given to me: she had attacked a member of staff and it wasn't possible to keep her at the home any longer.

There was a very different atmosphere in the home after she left. Staff and residents spoke of peacefulness. I noticed a silence where there had been singing and chatter. I missed Mrs G, I missed her spirit, her friendliness towards me. Her bed was kept open in case she could return, but she took a chest infection while in hospital, and died there.

8 | Reacting to a real threat

GRAHAM STOKES

At the root of Mrs O's "challenging" behaviour was a remembered threat still terrifyingly real to her. Once this threat was understood, from information gained through members of her family, an individual and unusual plan of care was devised which enabled her to relax and feel safe.

Mrs O is a 75-year-old woman suffering from a marked dementia of the Alzheimer type. Following the death of her husband several years earlier, she lived by herself until self-neglect and increasingly risky behaviour led to an admission into residential care. From the moment she entered the specialist dementia unit, she was a cause for concern. She was also a puzzle.

In daily life around the home she rarely displayed awareness of her surroundings. She spent much of the day sitting contentedly, often smiling at passers by, nodding and occasionally gesturing with her hand. She would participate passively in activities, and conveyed an aura of kindliness. Yet – profoundly forgetful, grossly disoriented and lacking meaningful speech – she also had high dependency needs.

Unfortunately, she reacted very badly to intimate care. At such times, she seemed transformed beyond recognition. Helping her out of bed, assisting her with dressing and washing were all met with unbridled ferocity. She was labelled unco-operative and violent, her behaviour dismissed as typical of advanced dementia.

It was her toileting difficulty, however, that caused greatest concern. Despite being inappropriately labelled by many staff as incontinent, she retained bladder control. She was rarely found wet in her bed or chair. Instead she would be observed walking around soiled. Staff would find wet clothing hidden away, and on occasions she would smear her bedroom or toilet. Helping her in the toilet, checking to see if she was wet, and attempting to change her clothing caused Mrs O great distress.

Her screams, abusive language and physical assaults on staff often degenerated into struggles. Two staff would invariably attempt to toilet her. This made the situation "manageable", but in no way reduced the trauma of the experience. Yet it was not her toileting difficulty that brought matters to a head. The catalyst for understanding was Mrs O's ulcerated legs.

Her leg ulcers had been a problem while she lived at home, and the district nurse regularly cleaned and dressed them. Mrs O appeared to have enjoyed these visits. Not only was there no record of distressed or uncooperative behaviour, but the notes documented how "chatty" and "jolly" she seemed. In the home, however, the senior care staff who now had responsibility for changing her dressings were met with the same distress observed during toileting. What had happened to the woman who enjoyed her one-to-one contact with the district nurse, whose reports also showed that she had taken Mrs O to the toilet with no difficulty? Why was it so different now she was in care?

The medical model offered a ready solution – dementia is progressive. Clearly she was now more demented than before, and thus more disorientated, disinhibited, and in general more difficult. Yet only a proportion of behaviour in dementia can be attributed to the presumed neuropathology.

Sensitive care was still not enough

Was Mrs O reacting to poor care practice? Not abuse or neglect, but insensitive care embraced by the term malignant social psychology? (Kitwood 1990). Observation revealed not. Care was sensitive and, when taken at face value, appropriate to her needs. Staff smiled, gently encouraged her to go with them and always offered a straightforward, paced explanation for their actions.

During intimate care they always promoted dignity and self-respect. For example, dressings would always be changed in the privacy of her bedroom; toilet doors would always be closed. Aware of the fragmentation of memory in dementia, staff would give frequent reassuring reminders of what they were doing and why. But this did not seem to help, nor did the non-verbal skills staff employed, such as eye contact, gentle tone of voice and comforting gestures.

The person discovered

Mrs O's only child, a daughter, visited the home regularly. As she came to trust staff, and overcame much of the guilt of seeing her mother in care, a picture of Mrs O slowly developed.

Her behaviour alarmed her daughter, for Mrs O had always been a morally upright, somewhat reserved woman. Her daughter had read about "disinhibition", yet found it difficult to reconcile her mother's abusive and hostile behaviour with the woman she had always known. She talked of her own strict upbringing, and her mother's overprotective attitude to her as a teenager, despite it being the "swinging sixties". She had grown to appreciate that her mother had a deep mistrust of men.

Mrs O had stayed at home until her marriage at the age of 30. Her husband was the local "man from the Pru". She was pregnant within a year, and seemed to exchange the closed home-centredness of life with her parents for the traditional role of wife and mother.

Mrs O's daughter rarely saw her parents being physically affectionate with each other, although her mother was demonstrably warm with her. Without ever enquiring or pinpointing anything of note, she gained an impression that her parents were not sexually intimate. There was the odd grumble from her father, an occasional snide comment and, of course, she was an only child.

Home life was unremarkable, despite there being a mysterious family schism. While there was regular contact with Uncle H, Mrs O's elder brother, they rarely saw her younger siblings (two sisters and a brother). Whenever they did meet there was tension in the air.

Uncle H still figured in his sister's life. He often visited the home, and regularly shed tears. Staff would see him holding her hand and would occasionally decipher the words "I'm sorry, pet". No other relatives visited.

One day I happened to visit the home at the same time as Uncle H. He had been particularly upset during his visit and staff had comforted him in a side room. They asked whether I would speak to him, and our conversation uncovered the motivation for his sister's difficult behaviour.

I had expected to be counselling a man distressed by the sight of advanced dementia. But he started to rebuke himself for letting his sister down, not standing by her when the others turned against her. He had always known that what she said was true, for he had been there. For years Mrs O had been subject to sexual abuse at the hands of her father. Uncle H had known about it; so had his eldest brother (killed during the Second World War). Their mother was protective toward her daughter, yet also colluded with her husband's abusive behaviour: she ensured that the matter was never spoken about.

The younger siblings never knew, and they loved their father. So when Mrs O, consumed with guilt and self-disgust, confided in her sisters, she did not receive understanding and compassion. They accused her of being malicious, and eventually ostracised her.

Why Mrs O was abused and not her sisters warrants only speculation. Uncle H did say their mother once had a friendship with a man who lived in an adjacent street, and who appeared especially fond of Mrs O when she was a young child. Could this be the explanation? A love child who became a figure of torment, and unwelcome reminder of infidelity?

The connection made

Nowadays residential care follows principles of home life. Staff rarely wear uniforms. Intimate care is practised within the privacy of a bedroom. There is very little in today's practice that is clinical or communal. Admirable developments, yet what were the implications for Mrs O? When her dressings needed to be changed she would be taken by a care worker, in her eyes a relative stranger, to the privacy of her room, sat on or by her bed, her skirt would be lifted and her stockings removed. In this setting, is it surprising that she feared what might happen next? Having lost reasoning and judgement, unable to recall, probably even understand the reassuring words of staff, and inhabiting a reality very different from ours but equally meaningful, meant that Mrs O now experienced her past in the present.

To be toileted was equally distressing: once again she found herself in a room where somebody was attempting to remove her clothes.

Person-centred solution

We decided to "medicalise" the dressings procedure. Mrs O had enjoyed the home visits from the district nurse not because she was less demented at that time, but because the situation was not threatening. The nurse turned up in her uniform with her bag and pursued the formal clinical procedure of dressing her leg ulcers. There was little chance for the mist of confusion to generate misunderstanding.

So the district nurse recommenced her visits to Mrs O. But rather than going to her room she was guided to the rarely used Treatment Room. Sat next to the medical trolley, cued into the clinical experience by an excess of bandages, dressings, ointments and forceps, the potential for misinterpretation was reduced. The space had an unambiguous, non-threatening use. (If recognition, recall and understanding have deteriorated, a design message must be made available through more than one of the senses. An example is a dining room where the clatter of knives and forks, the smell of food and the sight of crockery, dining tables and chairs all declare "this is where you eat". For Mrs O the outcome was a joy to behold. She was again that pleasant woman who sat in the chair and smiled. No trauma, no anger, just a fleeting peace of mind.

After a few visits from the district nurse, care staff again took responsibility for the dressings. We were uncertain whether staff out of uniform would again generate fears, yet we need not have worried. The sight and smell of the environmental cues gave the reassuring message "medical treatment".

Addressing Mrs O's toileting need was more challenging. Clearly, her toileting programme needed to encapsulate the lessons we had learned. She would never achieve assisted independence; her disorientation, aphasia and apraxia were too severe. Yet the privacy of the toilet, and the intimacy of care required, continued to upset her. Could we take advantage of the treatment room's anxiety-reducing cues?

A toileting programme of three-hourly visits was implemented. This fixed schedule required Mrs O to be taken not to the toilet, but to the treatment room. While sitting next to the dressings trolley, her keyworker would talk to and comfort her. It was not the contents of the conversation that was important, but the reassuring use of body language and voice tone. When soothed she would be taken across the room to where a commode had been placed behind a screen. Reassured by the abundant cues of the treatment room, Mrs O's behaviour gave evidence to how safe she felt. No anger, no violence. Instead, benign acceptance. There were still occasional outbursts, but these were few and far between, and tended to occur when staff tried to rush the procedures.

Conclusion

Mrs O is no longer seen as difficult. She is known to be frightened when her personhood is not acknowledged. A dementing person will select the manner of behaving which is appropriate in the light of how they interpret their experiences. What is deemed reasonable is, however, subjective, not objective. In Mrs O's case her traumatic history meant that staff had to accept that there are no set ways of working with a person who has dementia – just guidelines and intuition. This resulted in going against current thinking and introducing a programme of care that was reminiscent of past institutional practice. Yet it worked, for successful intervention is person-centred, not prescribed. With the subjective experience of dementia guiding our work how can it be otherwise?

Reference
Kitwood T (1990) The dialectics of dementia: with particular reference to Alzheimer's disease. *Ageing and Society* **10** 177-196.

9 ▍ Excluded from a role in the personhood club

JACKIE POOL

It was not Fred's wandering that concerned his son, but the underlying cause of it – a lack of meaningful occupation. The situation was leading to feelings of worthlessness and social withdrawal, denying Fred a sense of well-being. Jackie Pool describes the successful solution.

This is the story of Fred, an 85-year-old man whom I first met when he lived with his son. Fred had a moderate dementia and his son had contacted the consultant because he was having difficulty coping with his father's night time wandering and refusal to go back to bed. The consultant asked me to visit and assess Fred's level of cognitive and functional ability, so that I could work with his son to demonstrate ways of interacting with Fred which would enhance his well-being.

On my first visit, Fred's son explained that, for most of the time, his father was easy to look after, but that he could not do very much and spent a lot of time in his armchair looking at the television. The son was the sole caregiver. He described his relationship with his father as having always been difficult, and concluded by saying that all he really wanted was some medication which he could give to Fred when he became difficult.

When I first met Fred, he was sitting in his armchair. He did not turn his head as I entered the room and did not respond to my greeting. He gave all the appearance of a man with severe dementia. After explaining why I was there, I began to administer a standardised test of cognitive and functional ability. Initially Fred did not respond but then, slowly, he began to participate. The test uses a functional task , and Fred became more alert as he followed my directions. His score on this test indicated that he could not initiate actions to produce an end result. This finding confirmed Fred's unmet need.

Occupation – a basic human need

After writing a report of my findings I made an appointment to visit Fred and his son again to discuss the situation. I explained that Fred depended on others to enable him to carry out activities and they, assuming he was incapable of doing anything, had not been offering him this opportunity. Because he had nothing to do for so much of the time, Fred had begun to slide into complete withdrawal, only occasionally emerging to

assert his will by wandering and resisting attempts to return him to bed.

For Fred, the problem was not the wandering but the underlying cause of it: a lack of meaningful occupation, and therefore a lack of the feelings of self-worth, agency and social confidence which combine to give an individual a sense of well-being. Without the opportunity for occupation, Fred was also denied the chance to interact with others – occupation is a vehicle for social contact.

It is so important that we recognise the occupational nature of humans, and acknowledge that we all have a need or an urge to explore and master our environment (Kielhofner 1989). This urge motivates us to engage in occupations, involves us in interactions with the environment and in role performance in daily living tasks, in work and in leisure activities. Role performance is necessary to the maintenance of any social group. Therefore preventing someone from participating in occupation has serious effects: it excludes an individual from the "personhood club".

Being unable to have a role which is meaningful in society diminishes a person's perceived worth, to themselves and others, and sets an individual apart from the social group. This is a powerful explanation of why people with dementia become withdrawn, a state I have heard described as not "ill-being" but "non-being". In Fred's case he had ceased, in his son's eyes, to be productive, and therefore, to be.

Fred's return to being

Now we had identified the problem, a person-centred solution could be planned. Fred's son was interested in my definition of the problem, and willing to try a new approach with his father. So that his son could learn how to enable Fred to succeed in the performance of activities it was suggested that one of my assistants would visit once a week for 10 weeks. Fred and his son readily agreed to this.

The assistant used activities to demonstrate ways of breaking down tasks into achievable stages. She also demonstrated the power of good interactive skills, and how Fred could readily respond to the use of touch, an encouraging tone of voice, and validation of his feelings. In addition it was arranged that Fred could attend the day hospital once a week for more occupational therapy and to widen his social contacts. The same assistant who worked with him at home implemented the occupational therapy programme at the day hospital.

Fred was encouraged to talk about his interests and hobbies he had enjoyed in the past. He revealed an interest in football, telling us that he used to follow the local team with great interest. Fred had never had any particular hobbies, but had carried out the DIY tasks around the house. This knowledge was used to select appropriate media for the therapy programme.

A simple woodwork project to make a teapot stand was started – it involved sanding, gluing and constructing the component parts. Fred was guided to achieve this by verbal directions which broke down the task into stages involving no more than two steps. Praise and encouragement was regularly offered to reinforce Fred's achievements, which were viewed as remarkable by the son who had thought his father could do nothing.

At the day hospital Fred was encouraged to take part in some social group activities and also to spend some individual time with the occupational therapy assistant. He was encouraged to look at the sports page of the daily newspaper and the football was discussed with increasing vitality (and a definite bias towards the home team!) Fred was beginning to discover purposefulness and his self-confidence was returning.

Striking change

When I visited Fred again at the end of 10 weeks, he was again sitting in his armchair but this time he turned to greet me. It was striking how much more animated his face appeared, and there was a sparkle in his eyes. When I reintroduced myself, Fred reached for my hand and kissed it – what a wonderful expression of his well-being!

The time of the occupational therapy intervention was now at an end, but it was arranged that the assistant would hand over the information about her and Fred's work to a companion provided by social services, who would continue with an activity programme. Fred's son demonstrated that he now understood his father's level of ability, and that he had learned enabling techniques. The quality of the interaction between Fred and his son had improved. Conversation was now directed to Fred rather than over him. Fred was being included back into his

society. It seemed that, now Fred's son could view his father as productive, he was better able to relate to him. The son also reported that there had not been any incidents of the original perceived problem of Fred's wandering at night.

Of course, the relationship between Fred and his son has always been strained and a person-centred approach cannot work total miracles. There will be times when the therapeutic relationship between them cannot be maintained. However, the "companion" will help to maintain Fred's level of occupational performance and will continue to act as a role model of well-being, enhancing communication skills.

Interestingly, readministration of the standardised test at the end of Fred's therapeutic programme showed an improvement in Fred's cognitive function of one level. This indicated that he now could initiate actions to produce an end result. The impact of a person's state of being on the neurochemistry of dementia, and the subsequent neurological impairment is currently under investigation. Involvement with people like Fred helps us to gather the evidence of standardised tests for research studies into this phenomenon. This work is still at a very early stage: there may be many other variables which are present and contributing to the end result. The standardised tests of cognitive function are just one measure of evaluating the effectiveness of the work with Fred. The kiss on the hand gave equally meaningful, but far more graphic, information.

This case study is just one example of a person with dementia empowered to realise their potential for meaningful occupation – at the same time enjoying increased opportunities for interacting with others – who has become less withdrawn and begun instead to demonstrate feelings of well-being.

The importance of meaningful occupation must be recognised and given a higher priority than it currently attracts. This includes the need for training and education of all care-givers, and a commitment from managers and those who hold the purse strings, to allocate adequate resources to this work.

References

Kitwood T (1993) Person and Process in Dementia. *International Journal of Geriatric Psychiatry* 8 541-545.
Kielhofner G, Nicol M (1989) The Model of Human Occupation: a developing conceptual tool for Clinicians. *British Journal of Occupational Therapy* **52** (6) 210-214.

10 | A gentle way through the barrier of pain

CATHY CHATTEN

Elsie was imprisoned by her dementia in a world of chronic pain, and she seemed to have only two moods: withdrawal and hostility. Cathy Chatten recounts how imagination and sensitivity provided the key to her release.

A high pitched shriek shattered the peace of late evening. "Elsie's playing up again," commented my weary colleague, handing over the patients at the start of the night shift. Then came a knock on the office door – Elsie had bitten the nursing assistant who had been trying to help her to bed.

She had only been with us for a few days but already Elsie had established a notorious reputation. This 80-year-old lady's unpredictable and violent outbursts were at odds with her frail appearance, and we were at a loss as to the best way to care for her. Not only was she aggressive towards staff but she had been known to lash out at fellow patients. She also spent long periods sitting alone, quietly weeping.

We knew very little about her background: she had been discovered living alone in the kitchen of her rambling inner city terraced house. A music teacher, she had spent recent years caring for her parents and had never married. She was frail and unkempt, socially isolated and living in what could only be described as squalor. Her companions were the radio and a ginger cat.

She had no close family. A neighbour had alerted social services after he spotted her wandering around her garden on a winter's night, wearing only her nightie. Following her admission we hoped she could be placed in the community, but her "difficult" behaviour stood between her and most residential homes.

Withdrawn and hostile

It was my task as Elsie's primary nurse to assess her needs and devise a care plan that helped to bring out the best in her. This was a daunting prospect as she seemed to have only two moods: withdrawal and hostility. She reacted badly to most nursing interventions and was uncommunicative to say the least.

We try to embrace the philosophy of the new culture of dementia care when assessing people on our ward. I knew that we needed to look beyond "problem behaviour" and plan for longer term solutions that would improve Elsie's quality of life

and sense of well-being. But Elsie's isolation and hostility made it difficult to get to know her at all, let alone try to fathom out what made her tick.

Here was a lady with a seemingly profound degree of behavioural disturbance who had built a wall around herself, so impenetrable that it was hard to see how we could get through to her.

After she had been with us for a few days we decided that we really must establish a medical baseline. A very careful examination was carried out by a female doctor (instinct told us that Elsie might be marginally less resistive to another woman). This revealed a multiplicity of problems, including chronic arthritis in her joints and spine.

We could only speculate on how many years Elsie had suffered from pain, undiagnosed and untreated, and the distress it had caused her. The arthritis may also have been particularly compromising to her in her profession as a piano teacher.

This information gave vital clues to her behaviour. Pain is a highly subjective experience, fully known only to the person who has it. We might imagine that we know what another's pain feels like, but only the sufferer can say what it really means to them. A good definition of pain is that it is whatever the person experiencing it says it is. As professionals we should respond accordingly, but of course our judgment is often tempered by our own feelings of how severe the pain *ought* to be.

Elsie sat, imprisoned by her dementia in a world of pain that she could not communicate. To be in pain is bad enough, but what must it be like to be in pain and be ignored?

This was still only half the story, however. We now knew a little of Elsie's medical history but we needed to discover more clues to her behaviour. An agnostic approach was used, one in which we were willing to say, "I don't know why this lady behaves in the way that she does but I'm not going to label her as problematic until I've tried to find out why."

Planning care

We used the formula *Assess*, *Plan* and *Prevent*, followed by *Evaluate*, and put together a care plan for Elsie. The team made baseline assessments in the categories of mood, pain, continence and sleep. We also managed to find a niece who was able to give us some valuable biographical information about Elsie's personality and past.

It turned out that Elsie had always been a proud and independent woman, refusing help with the difficult task of caring for both parents in their last years, despite their increasing physical frailty. She was a devoted daughter and had put her parents before any thoughts of marriage and motherhood for herself.

She loved music, and it gave her great pleasure to help children learn to share that love, through the piano lessons she gave. Her taste was strictly classical; she did not appreciate "modern" styles such as jazz. She also had a great love of animals, particularly cats.

Elsie was not sociable by nature, her niece told us. All she ever really wanted was to be left alone in the house she had been brought up in, with her beloved cat and piano.

Here then was a lady who neither asked for nor wanted our help. Her problem behaviour was a reaction to the constraints of institutionalisation; there would not have been a problem in her own home. Sometimes in a hospital or residential care setting the baseline for an individual's behaviour is set artificially low. We cannot allow wandering where the environment presents a hazard, or disinhibited behaviour where there is no privacy.

We recognised this, yet felt that there was scope for Elsie's individual needs to be met with the right caring approach. The medical team had assessed Elsie's pain and prescribed analgesia, but we felt that other factors might contribute to her experience of pain. She was alone in a place she did not recognise, surrounded by strange, unfamiliar people, noise, and routines. Her confusion and difficulty in communicating increased her isolation. Once we started to look at life though Elsie's eyes we began to understand that she was protesting against life's injustices in the only way she could.

Developing trust

Through primary nursing, we encouraged consistency of care so that the number of unfamiliar faces Elsie had to contend with was reduced to a minimum. It took time to develop a bond with this frail and frightened lady, but eventually her aggression eased as she came to trust us. We made sure everyone knew that Elsie had painful arthritis and extra care was needed when carrying out nursing procedures. This measure in itself, over time, seemed to reduce the trauma Elsie experienced.

We also tried to de-institutionalise Elsie's experience of hospital. Information gathered from

the baseline assessments helped us to design Elsie's own personalised routine. She seemed to prefer to go to bed early and get up fairly early. She appreciated the peace and quiet of her own room, with a commode so that we could assist her in the night with minimal disturbance. In her own home she usually bathed in the evenings, according to her niece, so this was built into her night time routine whenever possible. During the day she seemed happier in the ward quiet room, away from the noise of the television and general hubbub.

The next step was to look even closer at Elsie's life history, if we were to successfully minimise the pain and distress that she was experiencing. We could not separate Elsie's pain and anxiety in looking at therapeutic approaches to her care, as they were closely interwoven. A therapeutic approach designed to reduce Elsie's anxiety would, we reasoned, have positive physical benefits. We worked with the occupational and physiotherapy departments to produce music, environmental and complementary therapy programmes for Elsie.

A musical life

Music was important to Elsie. It had always been there, in her work and in her leisure. Music had given her life colour, depth and texture, and her taste was as individual as her own life history. We used sensitivity and respect when making choices on Elsie's behalf. We did not always get it right.

We discovered that she preferred piano sonatas and string quartets, particularly the quiet second movements. The louder sections made her agitated, but soothing passages in chamber music relaxed her and very often sent her to sleep.

Creating the right atmosphere for Elsie's musical interludes was an important part of the therapy. Elsie enjoyed peace and calm around her, so we earmarked the quiet room and made sure that no-one disturbed her "time out". The lights were kept low and extraneous noise was kept to a minimum.

The only visitor allowed to disturb Elsie's privacy was Tigger, the ward cat (happily, ginger). Though normally preferring the linen cupboard to the ward, Tigger gravitated towards Elsie, spending hours curled up on her lap. Watching Elsie gently stroke Tigger, while she listened to soothing classical music, it was hard to imagine the terrified and hostile lady we had admitted only a few weeks earlier. Elsie also enjoyed quietly listening to the radio, just as she had done at home. When *The Archers* theme came on, Elsie's face positively lit up.

Elsie's "time out" was also used for complementary therapies. Our Trust does not have a policy allowing the use of complementary therapy as a treatment, but as a therapy we were able to use selected techniques. Elsie enjoyed "pampering sessions" – having her neck rubbed, having lotion gently applied to her hands – or selective, non-contact use of aromatherapy. What could be nicer than listening to soothing music, receiving a neck rub and enjoying the scent of lily of the valley around you?

These therapies, after a little initial trial and error, seemed to have a wonderfully soothing effect on this previously very disturbed lady. Sometimes, just sitting quietly with Elsie, holding her hand gently, seemed to magically drain the tension from her face. Consistency was the key to success. Elsie's "time out" was part of her day, just as essential as any other part of the care plan.

The rationale behind these therapeutic approaches was empowerment: they left decision and consent with Elsie, and were based on quality of life and enjoyment. We felt that in helping to meet Elsie's psychological needs in this way, she was encouraged to feel valued and comforted. She took a little while to respond, not surprisingly, but she was worth the investment. We saw her behaviour gradually become less disruptive, she needed less medication and slept better. Eventually she began to appear more sociable, taking an interest in other people on the ward, although she remained verbally uncommunicative. Staff picked up her non-verbal cues, however: Elsie gradually became more comfortable, more relaxed and more peaceful.

Not an optional extra

Sometimes, on a busy ward like ours, there seems to be so much that needs to be done that therapeutic approaches such as this may become low priority. For Elsie, however, therapies were not an optional extra but a vital part of her care. I believe that without a creative, individualised approach, we would never have tapped into the very real human need that lay behind Elsie's disturbed behaviour. This is the art of creative dementia care: looking beyond the behaviour to the person inside. Elsie was eventually placed in a small residential home that respected her need for peace and quiet, and had a sensitive approach to pain management. I am happy to say that they also had a friendly cat!

Protecting her personal source of love

DEBBIE CHRISTIAN

To engage with Ruby, it was necessary first of all to meet "person to person" with Toby: instinct led the author to make friends with the soft toy dog clutched in her new resident's arms. It was to prove a vital key to their developing relationship.

She swears.
She punches and pinches.
She tries to walk and falls over.
She needs to be sat in a reclining chair.
Is incontinent.
Is messy at mealtimes.
Cannot wash or dress herself.
Is resistive to care.
Is confused.

Who is this?

Ruby arrived on a bright, sunny spring morning bringing nothing with her but a Tesco bag of clothes, "Toby" (a small soft toy dog) and the above list of "nursing needs". She arrived at Mill House nursing home with no other introduction and introduced herself by giving a wry smile and landing a punch squarely on my chin in response to my cheery "Good morning".

With such an introduction, Ruby is in grave danger of never having the question "Who is this?" answered. Over a period of two years, she has been shunted between psychiatric hospital ward and nursing home, finally arriving at Mill House. Each previous placement has been a failure, because Ruby is a problem. Over the years, her identity, individuality, life history and uniqueness have been eroded to such an extent that she has become a list of behaviours. Even her name has disappeared from the language used to describe her.

Ruby has no recognised personhood. She is no longer viewed in the context of relationships and social being – merely as a set of behaviours with no implication of recognition, respect or feeling. Ruby is in desperate need of having her uniqueness and personhood re-established. Her identity and place in a social context requires reinforcement and her sense of agency (being able to make things happen) requires strengthening. What follows is an account and analysis of what Ruby and I achieved during the six months in which we knew each other.

Toby was the link

The starting point of our relationship was where I dismissed the labels attached to her, and made friends with Toby. Why I should do the first I understand, why I did the second so immediately remained a mystery to me for some time, but it proved to be the vital link in establishing our relationship.

When I first met Toby he was securely grasped in Ruby's arms, almost unidentifiable as anything but a ball of rags. The determination with which he was held so tightly to Ruby's chest and the incoherent mutterings she directed towards him aroused me to the fact that here was the thing Ruby treasured. I put out my hand, lightly touched his head and whispered, "Hello, who are you?" Immediately, Toby was clutched tighter. "It's Toby. Talk to Toby."

So Toby was shown into the home, introduced to others within it, and he and Ruby were made comfortable in their room. I then sat with Ruby as she shared her cup of tea with Toby and me. From that moment onwards, Toby became as real to me as he was to Ruby. I was able to engage in a relationship with Ruby because I discovered this passage into her world.

A relationship develops when personhood is recognised. When someone is truly treated as a person, meeting can take place. This meeting of persons involves a sense of equality and common purpose, openness, tenderness and awareness. To meet with Ruby it was necessary initially to engage "person to person" with Toby. By doing this, by lowering my barriers, perceiving and acknowledging Toby as Ruby did, I demonstrated respect and sensitivity to Ruby herself, entered into her subjective reality and made real contact with her.

As Ruby's keyworker it fell to me to assess her abilities and to devise her plan of care. If I had used quantitative assessment procedures, with measurements, scores and statistics, I would have discovered, as those before me had, the deficits in Ruby's abilities and skills. It would not have been difficult to see that Ruby had a core of problem behaviours, and to focus on these. The obvious danger is that Ruby as a person is ignored.

The purpose of any assessing I did was firmly rooted in the desire to answer the question, "Who is Ruby?" The focus of the next six weeks was getting to know her as she was, there and then. No amount of enquiry could elicit any life history about her. It appeared that she was important to no one and that her unique life history had been lost forever. But Ruby was there before me, real and unique and important to me.

Making choices, exerting her strong will

Ruby was well able to make choices; she expressed her wishes and desires both verbally and non-verbally, and if the person with whom she was interacting did not recognise or tried to deny her wish, she would forcibly exert her choice. For example, if Ruby was walking somewhat unsteadily around the home and a well intentioned member of staff, feeling she was unsafe, attempted to get her to sit down, Ruby would walk faster, struggle against any physical contact and hit out if staff persisted.

Ruby's ability to influence those around her and exert her right to make choices caused distress to care workers. They felt that Ruby was not able to make an informed choice and could not therefore understand the risk in which she placed herself. As "professional carers" they felt they had a duty to protect Ruby, and the only way they could do this was by denying her her choices. This attitude reflects the tradition of care which assumes that the person with dementia is incapable, requiring all things done and all decisions made for them. The focus of this tradition is control, management and medical treatment. It represents a failure to relate, an inability to enter into another person's world.

After long and heated discussions, staff began to recognise that Ruby experienced distress if she was denied her choices; that denying her the opportunity to walk freely about her environment caused Ruby a distress and state of ill-being that outweighed the risk she was taking. Care workers agreed that what they could do was ensure that Ruby wore correctly fitting footwear, that her immediate environment was kept clear of obstacles and hazards and that she be encouraged to walk using the aids available in the environment to assist her. They accepted that doing this would eliminate as many external risks as possible, without creating distress and ill-being for Ruby.

During the next six weeks Ruby had many falls, but always got straight back on her feet and set off again. Her confidence, her knowledge of her environment, her strength and stability increased,

and her falls decreased. Ruby had made her choice, and her well-being was enhanced by this choice being recognised.

Reframing the problems

Each of Ruby's "problem behaviours" was "re-framed" (looked at again from a different point of view) as in the above example. We sought to understand the "problems" as expressions of positive attributes in Ruby's character.

She swears. She punches and pinches. These actions were recognised as valid expressions of emotion; appropriate responses to situations and circumstances.

She tries to walk and falls over. This was Ruby being active and purposeful. Ruby always went somewhere and did something, no matter how small or inappropriate it seemed. Ruby was always "doing" – when we recognised this we were able to help her achieve small tasks to which she had been denied access before, such as tidying books and magazines, straightening chairs and re-organising drawers and cupboards.

She needs to be sat in a reclining chair. There are no such chairs at Mill House and Ruby never sat on one again.

Is incontinent. Cannot wash or dress herself. Is resistive to care. Ruby's continence improved with her increased mobility and knowledge of her environment. She retained a sense of self- respect and dignity. Given support and assistance in the sequencing of self care tasks, Ruby achieved a level of self care which required only re-assurance and assistance from care workers.

Is messy at mealtimes. Ruby always shared her food with Toby. When we provided an additional plate and portion of her meal for Toby too, Ruby's dietary intake improved and she stopped putting food on the table.

Is confused. Ruby used cues in the environment which enabled her to function appropriately within it. A large picture of Toby on her room door ensured that she always found her way home, and simple signs on other doors meant she always found what she was looking for.

This way of assessing Ruby recognised her unique strengths and qualities. It shifted the focus dramatically from "problem behaviours" to Ruby as a person able to express herself and make choices, and gave us some insight into her subjective experience of the world around her. Engaging in real meeting with others gave Ruby the opportunity to display great affection, humour and enjoyment.

Sparring partners

During the six months that I knew Ruby I discovered who she was, and also learned a great deal about who I am too. Ruby enjoyed a good, loud and aggressive argument. It could be about anything from not having enough sugar in her tea to protesting about the necessity of having a bath.

During these arguments, Ruby's features became more animated than usual and she would wink and giggle to onlookers who caught her eye. And when she won her battle she would wear such an air of smug satisfaction and gloat on her victory that it became an accepted part of daily life at Mill House that you argued with Ruby and that you always lost.

Some found this hard to accept and would not or could not engage in these battles of will, but to me it seemed that Ruby thrived on them and sought people out with whom she knew she could fight. I was one such person and spent many hours arguing with Ruby, both of us enjoying every minute.

It was said to me that I shouldn't be arguing with her; wasn't I denying her her sense of agency? Was I? I don't think so. I believe that I was meeting a need of Ruby's to engage in these verbal sparrings.

The need for love

Ruby taught me that love and comfort is a most necessary part of our everyday life and that its source, whatever or whoever that may be, requires nurturing and protecting. Ruby cared for and protected Toby with a fierce passion. She had been denied the love and comfort gained from human contact and had turned to Toby to both provide her with that love and also to fulfil the need in her to protect and nurture. (I can only surmise that Ruby once had a small dog called Toby.)

Ruby came to accept love and comfort from another source at the end of the time in which I knew her. She had a stroke, and while lying weak and frustrated in her bed, reached out to me and pulled me close until I was on the bed lying with her and just holding her tightly. Ruby drifted off to sleep but every time I tried to release my hold and move away, she gripped me more tightly and refused to let me go. She died lying in my arms.

Ruby showed me that the person is always there and that however hidden and masked it may be by other people's judgements and misconceptions, given the opportunity, a new light can always be shone on any situation.

Toby remains a part of my life and now lives with me. I must confess that he is not as well cared for as before, but he is still an extremely good listener...

12 | The gift of her friendship

MARIE MILLS

The close relationship and sharing of positive "person-to-person" experiences in good dementia care practice can bring benefits for the caregiver, too. This gift from dementia should not be underrated, and those who experience it should spread the word, writes the author.

I first met Amy in the autumn of 1990. A widow aged 80, she lived alone in a pleasant residential area on the outskirts of a market town. She had no children, and her next of kin was her only surviving relative, a younger brother aged 75, who lived 20 miles away. Amy's mild forgetfulness and confusion had become more noticeable after her husband's death in 1988. She had been brought to the attention of the psychogeriatric services in June 1990 by her GP where she was diagnosed as having moderate Alzheimer's disease. A very supportive community psychiatric nurse (CPN) was then assigned to monitor her progress in the community.

Her illness rapidly progressed and various worrying incidents caused her brother and the psychogeriatric services to consider the possibility of a move into residential care. I was approached and asked to assess her for our "befriending" scheme until a vacancy arose in our residential home.

Kitwood (1997) and Gilleard (1996) among others argue that community services for people with dementia must be adaptive. In this instance, as I provided the transport, the service was highly flexible and allowed the home to offer day care services in any format that suited the client. This could range from just having lunch to day care extending into early evening. So I rang the home help to arrange to visit when she would be there too, to introduce me to Amy.

I found Amy to be a sweet faced, kindly lady. She was welcoming on my arrival, and talkative; although she quickly lost the threads of conversation. Almost immediately she showed me around her home and commented on the contents of each room. This was to take place at most future meetings. It was as if Amy was reminding herself of her home and her belongings.

Sadly, much was being hidden, covered by cloths or stored in plastic bags in cupboards. This "putting away" from mind seemed to reflect the loss and desperate searching for control which is an inherent part of dementia (Kitwood 1990a, 1997; Woods 1989).

My initial, tentative assessment of Amy's needs was that she was lonely and needed more social contact. She also looked lost and anxious, indicating probable feelings of insecurity.

In a separate interview, her home help confirmed this assessment. She said that Amy was often reluctant for her to leave and seemed to be becoming "more frightened of life". Moreover, she was beginning to forget to eat and would wander around the neighbourhood.

It seemed, therefore, that Amy would benefit from some specialised and flexible day care. I invited her to visit us for lunch and she agreed. Initially this took place twice a week but was gradually extended to five days per week as her needs increased. The time spent in the home was also lengthened until eventually she was returning home in the evening. Assessment of this service took place on a regular basis with her CPN, home help, relative and myself.

A special bond

So began my relationship with Amy. But this is not entirely a story about assessment and meeting needs. Rather, it is an account of the pleasure we found in each other's company, together with the memories, which Amy helped to create, that are still vivid in my mind. Further, I would want to argue that these shared experiences have helped to create a bond which remains, even as cognition declines and speech fails.

Amy ultimately spent very weekday in the home. On Saturdays her brother and his wife would visit, and her home help prepared her meals on Sundays. We were on call for emergencies. She was always pleased to see me when I arrived to help make her ready for the day. This could often take some time as shoes and essential clothing would mysteriously disappear overnight. Her home help reported that this was not new behaviour. Eventually we would set off in the car. She would unfailingly remark on the weather and say that it was nice for April. She said that April was a good month because, "We know spring is coming." I always found this to be a hopeful comment, suggesting that she had not been overwhelmed by the malignant social psychology which so frequently accompanies the dementias (Kitwood 1990a).

On returning to her house we would frequently go via the town centre to do some shopping for the home or my own family. For Amy, every visit was seemingly a new experience. We would go to Marks and Spencer where she might choose a cake for tea. The cake was always a battenberg. As we wandered around the food hall she would marvel at the array of food and the colours of the fruit. She particularly liked the apples, perhaps because she recognised them more easily, and she would point out the many varieties.

When we approached the cake stand she would be amazed at the choice, and each wrapped cake was very gently examined. If she decided she would like one, there would be much hesitancy before making her predictable selection. After payment she would put it carefully away in her bag. When we reached her house I would help her put it on a plate, together with her sandwiches for later. At this stage of her illness she would forget to eat if food was not made visible.

Although I felt we were meeting her needs during her time with us, through "positive person work" (Kitwood 1997), Amy was beginning to wander from home in the day; either in the morning before I arrived, or on her return home after I had left. On several occasions she had been found lost and frightened. It is an anxious process monitoring someone's progress at home, especially for the first visitor of the day. It was decided at the following review that she would be at less risk of wandering from home if I called earlier in the mornings and she returned home when it was dark.

Thus, as Christmas approached, our visits to the town began to take place in the early evening. The streets were brightly lit with Christmas decorations and Amy would stand and exclaim with delight at the twinkling lights and rich colours. We would look in the shop windows and point out the most eye catching glittering decorations to each other. We also met people I knew who greeted us both and chatted to Amy. We visited a dress shop on a few occasions as Amy had been a keen dressmaker. She examined the garments hanging on rails and checked the quality of their seams, rubbing the fabric between her fingers thoughtfully. The staff were very kind to us and showed us sequinned party dresses and silky shawls.

Childlike joy

Emotion and memory have a strong association (Conway 1990, Mills & Coleman 1994, Mills 1997, Mills 1998) and my memories of these times are no exception. As I write I can recall feelings of wonderment – a childlike, but not childish, joy – and the pleasure associated with simple, safe and enjoyable activity. Probably, using Kitwood's (1997) concept of empathetic identification, I was identifying strongly with Amy at this point. These person to person experiences are powerful and long lasting, albeit "unlabelled" by the person with dementia. Amy has never remembered my name but has always recalled my face.

Day care continued until the middle of January 1991 when a single room became available. Amy settled quite happily into residential care, but after a few weeks she began to put herself to bed in a double room. We felt that she was lonely and was asking for the company of others. Her brother agreed and gave permission for her to share a double room with Hetty, a friend she had made. It was good to see them together. They would walk around the home holding hands, and go for walks together with members of staff. Amy was a great favourite with staff. Although her confabulated speech made understanding difficult, they found her gentle ways and laughter very endearing. Moreover, she loved to join in sessions of communal singing. Echoing the work of Bright (1992) her ability to sing her favourite songs remained unimpaired, and staff would listen to her cracked silvery voice and marvel at her recall.

Amy still remembered me and when I was near would often tug my clothes gently to gain my attention. She would say, "It's you, I know you!" This has continued until the present. I recall an exhausting day last year – the sort of day when one feels particularly ineffectual. Amy was walking down the corridor with her head bowed. I touched her hand and she looked up and immediately smiled. She laughed with enjoyment and said, "It's you!" I felt validated and, in a way, I too felt more secure. Her attachment to me felt positive and rewarding. There have been many such occasions.

Recently, Amy caught the flu. She was most unwell and it was thought that she might die. It is hard to lose residents who are close to us (Sutton 1997, Mills 1998). Moreover, it does not become easier with time. However, Amy slowly improved. Some weeks later, I found her dozing in the lounge in her recliner chair, covered by a brightly coloured crocheted blanket. i gently touched her cheek and she opened her eyes. Although she could not speak, her smile showed pleasure and recognition.

Meeting each others' needs

Amy's gift of memories, of shared "person to person" experiences, will not end with her death. She has shown that enjoyment, laughter and friendships are possible in dementia, with greater expression made possible through the new culture of dementia care (Kitwood & Benson 1995).

Further, Kitwood (1997) argues that the psychological needs of people with dementia cluster around the core concept of unconditional acceptance/love. These affiliated needs are concerned with comfort; the safety associated with attachment; the recognition that we are social beings through inclusion within the social group; the drawing on skills and ability through occupation, and finally, to have continuity with the past, to have a life story and to have identity. Kitwood (p84) maintains that meeting these needs in their entirety leads to a global sense of self-worth, of being valuable and valued.

I would suggest that these needs are also strongly present in those who care for people with dementia. In addition, the meeting of both participants' needs can be accomplished through the interactive processes associated with positive dementia care. Thus, people with dementia can reciprocate and are able to encourage their own carers to experience well-being. This gift from dementia should not be underrated, neither should it go unreported. Society, as a whole, has a tendency to focus solely on the negative aspects of dementia, although dementia care workers know that this is certainly not the whole story. Older people with dementia still have much to offer, but we are the only ones who can give an account of their gifts to us, whatever these may be.

References

Bright R (1992) Music therapy in the management of dementia. In Jones GM and Miesen BM (eds) *Care Giving in Dementia: research and applications*. Routledge, London.

Conway M (1990) *Autobiographical memory: an introduction*. Open University Press, Milton Keynes.

Gilleard C (1996) Community care: psychological perspectives. In Woods R (ed) *Handbook of the Clinical Psychology of Ageing*. Wiley, Chichester.

Kitwood T (1990a) *Psychotherapy and Dementia – Psychotherapy Section Newsletter* 8 40-56.

Kitwood T (1990b) The Dialectics of Dementia: with particular reference to Alzheimer's disease. *Ageing and Society* 10 (2) 177-196.

Kitwood T (1997) *Dementia Reconsidered: the person comes first*. Open University Press, Buckingham.

Kitwood T, Benson S (1995) (eds) *The New Culture of Dementia Care*. Hawker Publications, London.

Mills MA (1997) Memory, Emotion and Dementia, in Jones GM and Miesen BM (eds) Care Giving in Dementia Vol 2: research and applications. Routledge, London.

Mills MA (1998) Narrative Identity and Dementia: a study of autobiographical memories and emotions. Avebury Series, Ashgate Publishing, Aldershot.

Mills MA (1999) The Role of the Narrative in Dementia Care Work Reminiscence and Life Review Conference 1999. Selected Conference Papers and Proceedings, University of Wisconsin, 98-102.

Mills MA, Coleman PG (1994) Nostalgic Memories in Dementia: a case study. *International Journal of Aging and Human Development* 8 (3) 203-219.

Sutton L (1997)Out of the Silence: when people can't talk about it. In Hunt L, Marshall M and Rowlands C (eds) *Past Trauma in Late Life: European Perspectives on Therapeutic Work with Older People*. Jessica Kingsley, London.

Woods RT (1989) *Alzheimer's Disease: coping with a living death*. Souvenir Press, London.

13 | Haloperidol, hips and toenails

TRACY PACKER
MICHELLE JEFFERIES

At the age of 83, Mrs T had spent four months in three different wards recovering from a hip operation. Now awaiting admission to a local "EMI" unit, she was on "calming" medication which had the opposite effect so that she posed a huge challenge for staff. Without the drug Mrs T began to emerge as a person, and staff could begin a long but effective process of discovery and individualised care.

Mrs T arrived on our ward one summer day from a medical ward in the main hospital. She had been sent to await her place for admission to a local "EMI" Unit.

The ambulance crew came and went, leaving behind an elderly lady who was very agitated and distressed. Clearly frightened, she took a long time to respond in any other way, to either the staff or patients on the ward.

This transfer may have been a routine event for the team working there, but for Mrs T the implications were huge. At the age of 83, she had spent no less than four months in three different wards, recovering after an operation to repair her fractured hip. Yet again she was faced with the arduous task of trying to remember the routine, the people, the layout and all the many other details which hospital staff take for granted.

The nurse on the previous ward had passed on some information about Mrs T, describing her as a lady with vascular dementia who was not compliant with her daily care needs. She consistently refused help, including toileting, daily hygiene needs and dressing assistance. She had developed a urinary tract infection and constipation and was doubly incontinent. This had not been a problem before her admission to hospital. Her legs were swollen and painful, and she had been immobile for the most part since her hip operation.

She was prescribed haloperidol five times a day, with chloral hydrate at night in order to try and calm her down. This was not working.

Following a change in their admission criteria and role within the hospital, the team receiving Mrs T had only just begun to admit people with a dementing illness. Many of the staff were apprehensive, feeling de-skilled and lacking in knowledge about the care of this client group. Mrs T's responses to their care only seemed to reinforce those concerns; for many she represented their worst fears about working with people with dementia.

After a day or two Mrs T's continued non-compliance, and aggressive responses when receiving most care including feeding, began to cause staff considerable concern – not least because of the invariable screaming, kicking, scratching and biting which accompanied even the most minimal contact, and which was distressing for everyone involved or within earshot.

When her personal care needs were finally met, Mrs T would make an attempt to get around without using the walking frame provided. She had now begun to "furniture walk", teetering precariously between unstable chairs and tables, before sitting down on the nearest bed and folding other patients' clothes or "tidying" their cupboards.

As these people did not have dementia and could not understand her behaviour, they would often get angry with her or the nursing staff, who continually had to "take her away" and lead her back to her own bed area. This only increased Mrs T's determination to try again, which caused even greater frustration within the unit.

Highly demanding

At night time, despite regular doses of haloperidol and chloral hydrate, Mrs T became even more active and demanding of nurses' time. If she needed the toilet she would refuse to use the commode provided and urinate on the floor nearby. Sometimes she would even urinate on a nearby bed. She would frequently call out or attempt to leave her bed, as if she was afraid of being on her own in the dark.

The staff were concerned that she might fall and hurt herself, and had placed cot sides on the bed to try and reduce the risk. But this had made matters worse, as Mrs T would then try and climb over the top of them, or slide down the bed to get out at the bottom. This only increased the risk of a more damaging fall, or bruising and cuts on her delicate skin. Other tired and anxious patients were getting more and more irritable with her.

Things were getting worse and worse. Mrs T's

daughter (her only visitor) had become reluctant to come in and see her because she felt such visits only made her mother more distressed.

During the staff handovers in those first ten days, Mrs T's responses were discussed in detail. It was agreed that events could not continue in this way. The team agreed that key nurses needed to work with her at all times to build up a trusting relationship. Their main aims at this time were to maintain her safety while she was improving her skills at getting around, promote her independence as much as possible and try and alleviate her anxieties about contact with staff during direct personal care.

During these discussions the team concluded that Mrs T was highly independent and very sensitive about exposing any part of her body to other people, particularly during intimate personal care. She would not allow anyone to wash or dress her, and it was realised that she did not have any of her own clothes. She hated continence pads and refused to wear them, pulling them out and throwing them disdainfully on the floor or ripping them to shreds.

The team thought it was ironic that in her assessment on the previous ward the categories "Expressing sexuality" and "Self-esteem and dignity" had "Vascular dementia" written next to them. It was as if Mrs T could not be expected to have any self-esteem, dignity or sexual expression because she had dementia.

Mrs T's relationship with her daughter had also been severely restricted, and we felt this important link needed to be re-established. Staff began to contact the daughter regularly to keep her updated, and she was persuaded to bring some personal items of clothing in for her mother. We also discussed the use of cotsides and she consented to their removal, agreeing that the risks outweighed the benefits. She was also persuaded to bring in fruit and other "finger" foodstuffs to tempt Mrs T, who still refused to be fed at any time.

The situation appeared to relax for a day or two, until one morning after a distressing night, an episode of incontinence in her bed and yet another confrontational bedside wash, a tepid breakfast was thrown in disgust at the nurse trying to feed her. Then Mrs T kicked in the face the chiropodist who was trying to treat her feet.

By this time the team had called for some advice from a specialist dementia care nurse, who was undertaking some Dementia Care Mapping (DCM*) on the unit that day. Mrs T was just one of the people being observed, but in this instance the "map" was abandoned and Mrs T's care was discussed immediately. The member of trained staff learning about DCM was encouraged to think about and interpret what she saw.

Careful observation

Mrs T's fierce independence, her distress, her marked hand tremor (which had not previously been noted), and the "guarding" (protecting) of her hip had all been observed during the DCM. We thought it very likely that the tremor was a side-effect of haloperidol. If the tremor could be stopped, Mrs T would be able to hold cutlery and feed herself, assist in her washing and dressing, and use her walking frame. As it was, she could not even lift a small cup of tea to her lips without spilling the contents.

It also became clear she was experiencing pain in the hip which had been operated upon – and it was this side which the chiropodist had been attempting to treat.

The doctor was called to the ward, and the nurse in charge explained the situation. The haloperidol was stopped immediately, and suitable pain killers prescribed. These were given to Mrs T straight away. Other factors surrounding her care were discussed with the dementia nurse – for example the importance of finding out more about Mrs T's life before her hospital admission, and the need for nurses to give her social contact and attention at times other than during care tasks, in order to help rebuild her confidence in them.

The following morning, much to the amazement of the ward team (most of whom had been rather cynical about the withdrawal of haloperidol), Mrs T got out of bed, walked with her frame to the toilet, washed herself, dressed and ate a full breakfast. She was much more relaxed and even smiling at times. The tremor was still noticeable, but had significantly reduced.

Over the course of the next few weeks the team found out more about Mrs T, which helped explain much of her behaviour. For many years after her husband died she had lived on her own, refusing social services involvement of any kind, and never leaving the house alone. She had been, by her own admission at that time, phobic about being institutionalised. She had felt this way for over 30 years, although a reason for this fear was never fully established.

Through a stroke of luck we discovered that Mrs T had worked as head of the laundry at the local homeopathic hospital for 30 years. She recognised a nurse who used to work there, who recalled that Mrs T was very efficient at her job. This explained her preoccupation with other people's clothing. Once this was understood, Mrs T spent many industrious moments folding newly laundered bed linen for the staff, and sorting out piles of hospital nightwear.

Mrs T was also very particular about toilet seats. She would use a "proper" toilet, but even then would never sit down properly on the seat, no matter how clean it was. She would squat on her haunches and "hover" above the seat to use the toilet. Through trial and error staff learned that *any* attempt to make her sit on it properly would result in anger and distress. It was important that any new or temporary staff were told of this, rather than learning the hard way.

Mrs T would not sit on a commode under any circumstances, so it was removed and no further attempts were made to make her use it. Once her mobility began to improve, the inappropriate urinating ceased as long as she was able to use the main toilet.

Mrs T would also leave the toilet cubicle "mid-stream" if the member of staff left the area to give her the privacy that is normally valued. She would only complete her toileting needs if the staff member stayed in the cubicle with her, or talked to her continuously from outside the door. Either way, they could not go away even for a short time, or Mrs T would leave the cubicle partially undressed in a panic to find them.

This behaviour baffled the team, and no convincing explanation was ever found. Was she afraid of falling into the toilet? Had something nasty happened to her in a small enclosed space? What had happened had left her so terrified of being on her own? We never did find out, but at least a satisfactory compromise had been reached.

Mrs T's night time sleeping pattern never really changed, and she would still wander about looking for company or something to do. If this need was addressed, she would generally be quite quiet. If she had been able to use the toilet, she would sleep for four to six hours, which seemed to be enough for her. The team realised that if they pulled three of the four bedside curtains around her, rather like a small room, she treated that area as her own space.

Special attention

At about three-thirty in the afternoon, the noise of the children in the creche behind the hospital would make her agitated. She would talk about her need to take her children safely home from school. This maternal need was identified, and some members of the team took extra time to be with her during this part of the day, to talk about her love of children. Alternatively, she could often be seen walking arm in arm with a nurse who would be getting on with tasks that only need one arm free! Otherwise she would sit in the staff office and chat with the nurses while they completed administrative tasks.

It was discovered that she loved teddy bears, and took ownership of any stray soft toys that were left behind. One in particular stayed at her bedside at all times, and was a great source of comfort. She increasingly sought tactile contact with staff, most of whom responded well to this, although some found this aspect of her personality more challenging. Often she would spontaneously hug a person and then ask them to sit on her knee! This became a common sight.

Despite our efforts, Mrs T hated the shift changeover, as this meant her nurse for the day would go home. As a way of dealing with this, she would mask her worries in a joke. Her parting words to that person would be, "I'll throw you out of the window I will!" Perhaps this too arose from her need to have some control over the daily comings and goings.

Throughout this period, the team maintained regular phone contact with Mrs T's daughter, who was only too pleased to answer questions and receive updates about her mother's progress. We explained that her mother was now very affectionate, getting upset even when members of staff went home, and that we saw this as an understandable reaction probably indicating her need for stability. We reported that the distress was short lived, and now that staff knew more about Mrs T, less difficult to allay.

Towards the end of Mrs T's admission her daughter was eventually persuaded to come in and stay for longer visits, bringing with her chocolates and sweets. Mrs T was at her happiest and most relaxed at these times.

In November, Mrs T and her teddy bear were successfully placed in a nursing home. The information exchanged outlined all of her known foibles. No one wanted either Mrs T, her daughter, or other care staff to experience the trauma of learning the hard way, as they had done. The only thing the staff had not been able to do by this time, was to cut her toenails – not surprising, perhaps, after the episode with the chiropodist.

Four weeks later, just before Christmas, staff from the ward visited Mrs T in her new home to give her a Christmas present. They were overwhelmed with her progress. A well dressed, smiling Mrs T proudly showed them her bathroom, the photographs of her husband on their wedding day (she would never discuss him in hospital), and at long last, her newly cut toenails.